Breast Cancer & You

International Breast Cancer Treatments

INTERNATIONAL TOXICOLOGY, INC.
1998

International Breast Cancer Treatments
Worldwide Cancer Treatment Series

Michael L. Holcomb, Ph.D.
President/CEO of International Toxicology, Inc.
3846 Peppertree
Eugene, Oregon 97402
USA

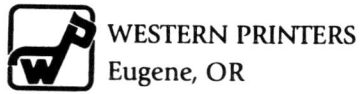 WESTERN PRINTERS
Eugene, OR

To My Mother

For Her Countless Encouragement

International Breast Cancer Treatments
Sponsored by
International Toxicology, Inc.
3846 Peppertree
Eugene, Oregon 97402

Sole distributor outside the United States
Copyright © 1998 by International Toxicology, Inc.

No copyright protection claim is made on materials "copied directly" from public domain materials of the United States or other governments.

All rights reserved. No copyright parts of this book may be reproduced or transmitted in any form or by any means, electronic or mechanical, including photocopying, recording, or by any information storage and/or retrieval system, without prior written permission from International Toxicology, Inc. Contact International Toxicology for information on foreign rights.

International Breast Cancer Treatments, this publication, is designed to provide a summary of the current treatment information for breast cancer in many countries. The research and treatments for breast cancer are advancing at a rapid rate. It is very important that patients contact the appropriate medical professional to determine the right treatment for breast cancer. All countries regulate the types of treatments allowed in their regions of authority. Thus, treatments allowed in one country may not be legal in another country.

This document is intended to collect information on breast cancer treatment worldwide. The more information a person has on the subject will allow for a better decision.

This book is sold with the clear understanding that the author and publisher are not engaged in giving medical, legal, treatment, or other professional advice or services. Absolutely no responsibility is assumed by the author or publisher for any injury and/or damage to humans or any other legal body in any event for incidental or consequential damage in connection with, or arising out of, the furnishing of this information. The author and publisher make no warranty of any kind, expressed or implied, with regard to the information contained in this book.

ISBN: 0-9644990-3-7
Library of Congress Catalog Card Number: 97-78275
Printed in the United States of America

Cover Design: Michael Holcomb and ProtoType

TABLE OF CONTENTS

CHAPTER 1: INTRODUCTION 7
1. Primary Ways to Get Cancer 7
   Genetic Inheritance 8
   Exposure to Human Carcinogens 8
   Other, Lesser Known or Unknown Factors 8
   Unknown Factors 9
2. Secondary Ways to Get Cancer 9

CHAPTER 2: BREAST CANCER TREATMENT .....
IN THE U.S.A. 11
1. How to Detect Breast Cancer 12
   Breast Self-Examination 12
   Clinical Breast Examination 13
2. Breast Cancer Treatments 14
   Surgery 14
   Chemotherapy 14
   Radiation Therapy 16
   Endocrine Therapy 16
   Clinical Trials 17
3. Diagnosing Breast Cancer 18
   Staging Breast Cancer 18
4. Progress Against Breast Cancer 25
   New Attitude 25
   BRCA Genes 26
   Other Genetic and Risk Factors 28
   Possible Risks 29
   Anatomy of a Disease 31
   Progress in Therapy 33
   Treating Early-Stage Disease 34
   Tamoxifen 36
   Treating Advanced Disease 37
   Determining Therapy 38
   Mammography: A Life-Saving Step 40
   Breast Self-Examination 42

Reconstruction Options 43
Implant Placement 44
Definitions of Breast Cancer Terms 47
What's New in Breast Cancer Research
   and Treatment? 53

CHAPTER 3: WORLDWIDE LEARNING 59
Europe 59
Germany 60
Italy 61
Japan 61
Canada 62
France 62
United Kingdom 63
India 64
Spain 65
Former Soviet Union 65
United States of America 65

APPENDIX 79
Chemotherapy and You 81
Radiation Therapy and You 117

Index

Chapter 1
Introduction

The treatments used to fight breast cancer worldwide are included in this book. While we have attempted to collect as much treatment information as possible within our timeline, obviously some methods are missing from this first volume.

The goal of this publication is to provide breast cancer treatment information on a global scale. This first volume is our initial installment on this goal. We believe that the best way to fight cancer is to be aware of the "weapons" (treatments) that are available worldwide.

There are many books on breast cancer and its treatments, but we are unaware of any books that attempt to view breast cancer treatments and mechanisms of action from an international perspective. Worldwide the definition of cancer is roughly the same. Cancer is the uncontrolled growth of cells that can be non-invasive (benign) or invasive (malignant). While there are many theories, hypotheses, and assumptions on the mechanism of cancer, none provide the ultimate cure. However, it is my opinion that there are only three primary ways to get cancer, a few secondary ways, and lots of combined primary and secondary ways. Now that you are thoroughly confused, let me explain. We created the terms primary and secondary ways to simplify the issues.

PRIMARY WAYS

The primary ways to get cancer are the ways that give a

person the highest possibility of getting cancer. Based on my scientific literature review, the primary ways to get cancer are: 1) genetic inheritance; 2) exposure to human carcinogens (chemicals); and 3) other, lesser known and unknown factors.

Genetic Inheritance

The genes play a major role in biological expression. What is not clear from the scientific research and literature is whether it is the recessive or dominant gene expressed in an offspring that insures a biological expression of all cancers. What I am certain of is that some types of cancers are inheritable. While the sex link gene may play a vital part in certain types of cancer, it is unclear what has to occur for the cancer expression to show up in the child (offspring). It is my opinion that cancer, if inheritable in a sex link fashion, must be dominant if it is expressed in all offsprings of the same sex. Why? My rationale for this conclusion is if the male provides any recessive or dominant gene to the female offspring, the outcome would still result in cancer for 100% of the females born into a family.

Exposure to Human Carcinogens

The scientific data are clear that exposure to known human carcinogens result in cancer to the exposed individual and/or the offspring (children). It is my opinion that women should never be exposed to any chemicals that cause birth defects, unless the person has passed child-bearing age and the chemical has no significant biological effect on the person being exposed.

Other, Lesser Known or Unknown Factors

Lesser Known Factors: The lesser known factors are the roles viruses, bacteria, parasites and nutrition play in cancer. It is obvious that a well balanced diet is important in maintaining good health. The acute effects of a poor diet will most certainly be of a significant concern more than the long-term possibility of cancer. What I am saying is that if a person does not eat a well-balanced diet, her diseases are likely to cause a significant possibility of death, e.g. heart disease, then cancer. But the important role of nutrition cannot be underestimated.

The roles of pathogens like viruses, bacteria and parasites, in inducing cancer is not well understood. But they may play some role to a lesser extent in producing cells or stimulating cells that can lead to cancer.

Unknown Factors: The amount of information we do not know about cancer outweighs the total sum of information we know. There are unknown factors that influence the growth of cells. For the last 20 years these unknown factors have continued to cause personal mental pain. For if we knew what turns a cell on, we could turn it off. But now we must kill both good and bad cells in an attempt to save human life.

SECONDARY WAYS TO GET CANCER

The environment that we live in provides many potential opportunities to come in contact with both natural and unnatural cancer-causing agents.

Exposure to excessive radiation from the sun both intentionally and unintentionally can result in certain types of cancer. Radon exposure in homes and other natural sources of radiation can lead to cancer. Inhaling secondary smoke, excessive drinking, and other habits can lead directly or indirectly to getting cancer. The secondary ways to get cancer are the ways that are sometime not in a person's immediate control, but can impact the health of those being exposed.

While I have attempted to simplify the many ways cancer can be initiated, it is important to note that cancer is a complex cellular response to many factors. It is equally as important to note that many treatments have been developed to deal with cancer. Where there is hope, there is life, and many people with cancer are alive today because of the great successful treatments and preventative measures that are now in place to deal with cancer.

Keep the faith.

Chapter 2

Breast Cancer Treatment in the United States of America

Breast cancer in the United States of America (and in all other countries) is a tumor or group of cells that has developed from cells in the breast(s). The breasts are classified as glands that are located below the neck on the front chest wall. All cancerous cells are characterized by abnormal, out-of-control growth. These cells can disrupt normal body tissues and organ functions. Not all breast tumors are cancerous. Not all lumps in the breast are tumors.

Breast cancer occurs most frequently in women and rarely in men. The American Cancer Society estimates for 1997 about 44,190 deaths from breast cancer in the United States.

Breasts are more developed in women because of hormones. Estrogens are responsible for breast duct development and progesterone for the development of the lobules.[2]

Human female breasts produce and release milk in association with pregnancy. The breasts are composed of milk-secreting glands, ducts, fatty, connective, and lymphatic tissue. The glands of women's breasts that can produce milk are lobules. The small passages connecting the milk-producing glands or lobules to the nipples are ducts.

One of the most important things we learned while writing this book is the importance of early detection of breast cancer. The earlier the breast cancer is detected, the higher the possibility of a complete cure. In most cases, nearly the entire breast can be conserved (saved) minus the cancerous tumor and some surrounding health tissue.

HOW TO DETECT BREAST CANCER
Breast Self-Examination (BSE)

A powerful tool women can use to detect breast cancer is the BSE. While this exam is not a substitute for an excellent doctor or routine mammogram, it does help in early detection. An estimated 80 per cent of breast lumps are not cancer, but the doctor should be made aware of your lump. BSE is recommended a few days after the menstrual period. The breasts are expected not to be tender or swollen a few days after the menstrual period.

Post-menopausal women should examine their breasts on the same day each month.

BSE is public-domain material. Please share this information with all interested individuals.

Examine Your Breasts Each Month

A. Looking: Stand in front of a mirror with the upper body unclothed. Look for changes in the shape and size of the breast and for dimpling of the skin or "pulling in" of the nipples. Any changes in the breast may be made more noticeable by a change in position of the body and arms. So, look for any of the above signs or for changes in shape from one breast to another.

1) Stand with arms down.
2) Lean forward.
3) Raise arms overhead and press hands behind your head.
4) Place hands on hips and tighten chest and arm muscles by pressing firmly inward.

B. Feeling: Lie flat on your back with a pillow or folded towel under your shoulders and feel each breast with the opposite hand in sequence. With the hand slightly cupped, feel with flattened finger tips for lumps or any change in the texture of the breast or skin; also, note any discharge from nipples or scaling of the skin of the nipples. Feel gently, firmly, carefully and thoroughly. Do not pinch your breast between thumb and fingers. This may give the impression of a lump that is not actually there.

1) Place a pillow or folded towel under your left shoulder. This raises the breast and makes examination easier. Place your left arm over your head. With your right hand, feel the inner half of your left breast from top to bottom and from nipple to breastbone.
2) Feel the outer half from bottom to top and from the nipple to the side of the chest.
3) Pay special attention to the area between the breast and armpit itself.
4) Now, place the pillow or folded towel under your right shoulder. Repeat this same process for your right breast using the fingers of your left hand to feel.

If you find something which you consider abnormal, contact your doctor for an examination. Most breast lumps are not serious, but all should come to the doctor's attention for an examination and a medical opinion. You may have a condition that will require treatment or further study. If necessary, your doctor may recommend laboratory tests or x-rays as part of a more detailed examination. Keep up this important health habit even during pregnancy and especially after menopause because the likelihood of breast cancer increases with age.

Clinical Breast Examination

Trained health professionals are able to conduct breast examinations. The American Cancer Society recommends that women the ages of 20 and 39 have a clinical breast examination every three years. Obviously, if you detect anything unusual during your BSE, see a doctor. Women after age 40 should have a clinical examination every year. Women aged 40 and older are in a higher risk group and may elect to have a screening mammogram.

[End of public domain material.]

BREAST CANCER TREATMENTS

There are four primary treatments for breast cancer in the United States. The treatments are surgery, chemotherapy, endocrine therapy, and radiation therapy. The type of treatment depends on the stage of development of breast cancer. Also, a combination of two or more of the treatments can be used.

Surgery

Surgery involves procedures to remove the tumor, some surrounding healthy tissue, or the entire breast(s). Samples of lymph nodes under the arm may be taken. Certain terms are used to describe the extent of surgery.

Local Therapy involves a variety of surgical procedures to remove the tumor and varying amounts of surrounding tissue and may include radiation treatment.

Lumpectomy is the removal of only the tumor (lump) and a rim of normal tissue. A few lymph nodes under the arm may be removed and examined for cancer. In general, lumpectomy is almost always followed by radiation therapy.

Partial or Segmental Mastectomy or Quadrantectomy: The removal of up to one-quarter or more of the breast. The axillary lymph nodes under the arm may also be removed. Radiation therapy is commonly used following surgery.

Simple or Total Mastectomy: The removal of the entire breast.

Modified Radical Mastectomy: The removal of the entire breast and axillary lymph nodes.

Radical Mastectomy: Very extensive removal of the entire breast, axillary lymph nodes, and the chest wall muscles under the breast.

Chemotherapy

The use of drugs in the treatment of breast cancer is called chemotherapy. Some drugs used in the treatment of cancer are toxic to both healthy and cancerous cells. Drugs that kill cells are considered cytotoxic.

The best way to get information on the drug(s) used in a patient's specific treatment is to ask the attending physician to describe specifically how the drug(s) work. The Physicians Desk Reference and the American Cancer Society can provide additional information on new treatments. Some cytotoxic agents work better together and can be used as a combination in the treatment of breast cancer. For example, cytoxan, methotrexate, and 5-fluoruracil can be used in combination to treat breast cancer.[3] The way these drugs work, or the mechanism of action, is complex. 5-Fluororacil (or fluorodeoxyuridine) is converted in the body into fluorodeoxyuridylate 5. The metabolite, fluorodeoxyuridylate, looks like a naturally occurring chemical the body normally uses (2'-deoxyribouridine monophosphate) to make nucleotides.[4] The metabolite irreversibly stops (inhibits) thymidylate synthase. The bottom line is ultimately the cell cannot function because it cannot make the appropriate nucleotide. Cancer cells grow so fast they need deoxythymidylate to make the building blocks of life (deoxyribonucleic acid or DNA). Fluorouracil, when metabolized in the body, prevents the production of deoxythymidylate. Methotrexate stops the making of deoxythymidylate which is needed to make DNA.

Before a new drug can be legally used in the United States, it must be approved by the United States Food and Drug Administration of the Department of Health and Human Services.[5] New anti-cancer drugs are being developed at a fast rate. From a toxicologist's perspective, these drugs are extremely toxic to both healthy and unhealthy cells. The risks and perceived benefits from the use of these drugs must be closely considered.

Chemotherapy Risks and Benefits

The risks and benefits of chemotherapy agents sometime become equal. For example, the chemotherapy agent L-phenylalaine mustard can be used as an adjuvant chemotherapy agent in the treatment of cancer, but may increase the possibility of leukemia in the patient.[6] Trading one type of cancer for another type of cancer is not necessarily a good situation.

The short-term, acute side effects of chemotherapy agents depend on which drug or combination of drugs is used in the treatment program. The word "side effect" describes the undesirable reaction that a drug can cause. The most common side effects are nausea, vomiting, hair loss (alopecia) and fatigue.[7] A reproduction of the public domain, free publication provided by the National Institutes of Health on *Chemotherapy and You* is in the appendix of this book. This booklet provides an excellent overview of chemotherapy. The pictures are not included in our reproduction. Please notice we have not altered this material because it is most valuable in its reviewed form. However, we have made notes where we are aware of changes in the information that is available.

The best way to weigh the risk and benefits of the specific drug(s) one may consider in chemotherapy is to have a conversation with the medical professional attending your case. If you cannot have these types of discussions, it may be wise to have someone who can represent your concerns or questions.

Information is power, and you should seek the answers to the questions you have about chemotherapy before taking on this treatment.

Radiation Therapy

Breast cancer can be treated with radiation, including x-ray, electron beam, alpha and beta particles and gamma rays. The use of radiation in the treatment of breast cancer is called radiation therapy. Radiation at very high levels can kill breast cancer cells. Radiation can be applied directly to the cancer cell (intraoperative radiation) or externally.

The instrument used to give radiation treatment is sometimes overwhelmingly large. Do not fear the machine. It is designed in this way to provide the most accurate method of positioning the treatment on the cancerous cells. The National Institutes of Health provides a booklet called *Radiation Therapy and You* that describes the treatment of cancer with radiation. We have reproduced this public domain publication for your benefit. (See the Appendix.)

The total effects of radiation therapy are not known, but the immediate help it can provide against cancer is known. Until a "cure" for cancer is found, radiation therapy will remain an important tool in the fight against cancer.

Endocrine Therapy

Some breast cancer tumors require the estrogen hormone

to grow. Chemicals that look like the estrogen hormone, but do not give the same growth response, are used to treat estrogen-dependent tumors. Think of it like this: There are two twins, one named estrogen and the other named anti-estrogen. They both would like to use the family car. If estrogen gets the car first, there will be a party and lots of growing friends will come (tumor formation). If anti-estrogen gets the car, the doors will be locked and no party will be held (anti-tumor). If you have ever had to compete with someone for a car, it is better to have an edge (the keys).

The dose of anti-estrogen is reasonably high and allows it to get to more sites. Technically, estrogens and anti-estrogens both compete for the estrogen receptor. Anti-estrogens like tamoxifen can bind to and translocate estrogen receptors to the nucleus.[8] The normal cell activities cannot be completed, and this influences a decrease in tumor growth. An estimated 35 percent of breast cancer in premenstrual women is estrogen dependent.[9]

Tamoxifen is given orally and affects many areas of the body including the estrogen-dependent tumor. Tamoxifen can hurt the fetus. Patients receiving adjuvant tamoxifen therapy should be aware of the potential side effects. Cardiovascular disease was shown to increase in women older than 60 years.[10] Some scientific data suggest tamoxifen increases uterine cancer (endometrial cancer).

Clinical Trials

The myth that people are used as guinea pigs in experimental programs to treat disease may prevent people from volunteering for clinical trials. In the days before strict regulations were put into place, this myth may have been closer to truth. But today valid medical research studies are designed to answer scientific questions that will help prevent or cure cancer. A volunteer must be given the details of the study in terms that are clearly understandable. Most importantly, you can choose not to be part of a clinical trial or leave a trial if it is not meeting your expectations. Readers can find out more information on clinical trials on the Internet. A few Internet sites on breast cancer may be helpful. Please remember to verify the information you read on the Internet. While the

Internet can provide sound scientific information, there is a lot of "junk" on the Internet that is not sound or true.

For breast cancer clinical trials, see the website at http://www.nabco.org.

Patients will have to be screened before they can enter clinical trials. Your doctor will be able to assist you in selecting a trial if it is appropriate.

DIAGNOSING BREAST CANCER

The American Cancer Society suggests that early measures are taken to detect breast cancer. Self-exam, clinical breast exam, consulting a specialist, mammography and ultrasound are the essential tools of early detection.

Recently, two genetic mutations, BRCA1 and BRCA2, were identified with inherited breast cancer.[11] Women who have close relatives who have had breast cancer can be tested for these mutations to determine their potential risk of getting breast cancer.

Once a lump is located, a sample of the lump may be taken (biopsy sample) to determine the stage of the cancer. The doctor will select the method of biopsy. The current types of biopsies are fine needle aspiration, core, and surgical. According to the American Cancer Society most health professionals prefer a "two-step" biopsy. The procedure can be performed in the doctor's office or hospital outpatient department. If cancer is detected, the second step, the appropriate treatment, can be taken at a later time.

STAGING BREAST CANCER

A systemic method used to determine the extent of the spread of the cancer is called "staging." The American Cancer Society describes staging as the following*[Public domain materials]*:

How is Breast Cancer Staged?

Staging is a system that uses information learned about the tumor through the diagnostic process to tell the doctor how widespread the cancer is. Thus, if cancer is detected by a biopsy procedure, additional tests will probably be done to determine the stage of the disease. The stage of a cancer has a great deal of impact on what treatment is selected. The cancer care team should be asked to explain the stage of the cancer so that the woman can make fully informed choices about her treatment. Following is a brief review of the various stages.

Lobular carcinoma in situ (LCIS): While not a true cancer, **lobular carcinoma in situ,** sometimes called **lobular neoplasia,** is classified as a condition signifying greater risk of developing breast cancer. In situ is a term used to indicate an early stage of cancer in which a tumor is confined to the immediate area where it began. In the case of lobular carcinoma in situ, the condition begins in the milk-producing glands, but does *not* penetrate through the wall of these lobules. Most researchers think that LCIS itself does not usually become an invasive lobular cancer, but women with this condition are at increased risk of developing an invasive breast cancer elsewhere in the same breast or in the opposite breast later. Studies are currently underway to help define the most appropriate way to deal with this increased risk. For this reason, it's important for women with LCIS to have a physical exam two to three times a year and an annual mammogram.

Stage 0: Ductal Carcinoma in Situ (DCIS): This condition is a cancer at the earliest stage that breast cancer can be diagnosed. In DCIS, there are cancer cells located in a duct, or milk-carrying passage, that have not escaped into the surrounding fatty breast tissue. Nearly 100% of women diagnosed at this stage can be cured. Changes caused by DCIS can usually be seen on screening mammography. With more women getting mammograms each year, this diagnosis is becoming more frequent.

Stage I: At this stage, the tumor is less than 2.0 cm (about 3/4") in diameter and does not appear to have spread beyond the breast.

Stage II: In Stage II, the tumor is either larger than 2.0 cm (about 3/4") in diameter or has spread to the lymph nodes under the arm on the same side as the breast cancer, or is both larger than 2 cm *and* present in these lymph nodes. In Stage II, the lymph nodes are not attached to one another or the surrounding tissues.

Stage III: This is a more advanced breast cancer which has spread to lymph nodes under the arm. The tumor is either larger than 5 cm (over 2") in diameter, or the lymph nodes are fixed (attached) to one another or surrounding tissue or both of these findings are present. Staging studies show no signs that the cancer has spread to distant organs or bones.

Stage IV: This stage indicates that the tumor, regardless of its size, has metastasized (spread) to distant organs. Even with metastatic disease, women with breast cancer may live for many years.

Remember that a variety of treatments are available for cancers in each of these four stages. No matter at what stage a breast cancer is diagnosed, a woman should be sure to discuss all options for that stage with her health care team.

The Staging System of the American Joint Committee for Cancer Staging, as just reviewed, is sometimes also known as TNM system of staging breast cancer. It uses the letters "T" for tumor size, "N" for extent of spread to lymph nodes, and "M" for distant metastasis (or spreading). Once a specific tumor has been staged using the TNM system, the TNM stage can be applied in a process called stage grouping which ranges from Stage 0, the least serious or earliest stage of cancer, to Stage IV, the most serious or advanced stage.

How is Breast Cancer Treated?

In the last two decades, considerable progress has been made in the treatment of breast cancer. Treatment, and the range of options available to the patient, are highly dependent on the type and size of a tumor and on how far the breast cancer has progressed at the time of diagnosis. The process of determining type and size of the tumor and how far it has progressed is called staging.

We will first discuss **treatment options by stage** of the cancer. Then we will review details of each option, including side effects. This review is intended to help explain the various treatments so the patient can discuss them with her health care team. Each patient has a different set of findings, and the health care team will discuss their specific recommendations with the patient.

In Situ Breast Cancer

In situ means that the abnormal cells are confined to the area in which they first appeared and have not spread.

Lobular carcinoma in situ (LCIS): Although LCIS is often classified as a type of breast cancer, most researchers feel it is better considered as a pre-malignant (pre-cancerous) condition predicting increased risk for developing breast cancer. Sometimes this condition is called **lobular neoplasia.**

Treatment Options for LCIS: Treatment usually involves only continued observations with follow-up physical exams and mammography. In exceptional cases, a bilateral simple mastectomy (removal of the breast) may be done. The surgery may or may not include reconstruction to restore normal appearance. Since LCIS puts a woman at higher risk for developing an invasive breast cancer in either breast, it warrants regular follow-up. While additional therapy may not be recommended, women may wish to consider participating in a clinical trial for breast cancer prevention.

Stage 0—Ductal Carcinoma in Situ (DCIS): This type of in situ breast cancer arises in the milk-carrying ducts of the breast and is biologically different from LCIS. DCIS is the earliest stage at which breast cancer can be diagnosed. In DCIS, the tumor cells are confined within the ducts of the breast and have not yet invaded the surrounding tissue. These tumor cells can become invasive over time without treatment. In contrast with lobular carcinoma in situ (LCIS), the invasive cancers that develop after a DCIS diagnosis tend to occur in the same area of the breast where the DCIS was first diagnosed. Nearly 100% of women diagnosed at this stage survive five years or more. Changes caused by DCIS can usually be seen on screening mammography.

Treatment Options for DCIS: Treatment options include removal of the breast tissue containing the DCIS, either with or without radiation. There also may be simple mastectomy (removal of all of the breast), with or without reconstruction. The axillary lymph nodes under the arm are not removed unless the size of the DCIS is quite large.

Invasive Breast Cancer

Stage I: In Stage I, the tumor is 2.0 cm (about 3/4") or less in diameter with no spread to the underarm (axillary) lymph nodes.

Treatment Options for Stage I: One option is a lumpectomy (removal of the lump only) or partial mastectomy (removal of a larger part of the breast) with dissection of the axillary lymph nodes under the arm, followed by radiation. Another option is modified radical mastectomy (removal of the breast and lymph nodes), with or without reconstruction to restore normal appearance. In addition, if the tumor is limited to 1 cm (less than 1/2" inch) in diameter, no systemic therapy is required. However, for some women, participation in a clinical trial to determine the best treatment is a possibility. If the tumor is larger, and depending on its specific features, the health care team may suggest the addition of chemotherapy or hormonal therapy, or both.

Stage II: In Stage II, the tumor is over 2.0 cm (3/4" in diameter), and/or has spread to the axillary (underarm) lymph nodes which remain movable.

Treatment Options for Stage II: Surgery and radiation treatment options are the same as for Stage I tumors, but systemic therapy likely will be required, depending upon whether the axillary lymph nodes are positive or negative for cancer. If the nodes are negative, recommendations may range from no systemic therapy, to chemotherapy or hormonal therapy, or both. If nodes are positive, chemotherapy or hormonal therapy, or both, are indicated. If there are several (usually ten or more) positive nodes, a woman in excellent health may choose to participate in a clinical trial of high-dose chemotherapy with stem cell or bone marrow transplant.

Stage III: In Stage III, the breast cancer is more advanced with the tumor larger than 5.0 cm (2 inches) in diameter and/or involving lymph nodes under the arm which are attached to one another or adjacent tissues.

Treatment Options for Stage III: This stage is divided into two parts, IIIa and IIIb. Because of the advanced nature of this stage of breast cancer, more aggressive treatments are required. For IIIa, there may be preoperative chemotherapy, followed by modified radical mastectomy, with or without reconstruction, and radiation. For IIIb, which includes cases of inflammatory breast cancer, the options are preoperative chemotherapy, modified radical mastectomy and radiation or, in some cases, radiation without surgery. In terms of systemic therapy, in IIIa, chemotherapy is usually given during pre-and post-surgery with or without hormonal therapy. In IIIb, systemic therapy may include chemotherapy both pre- and post-surgery, with or without hormonal therapy, and clinical trials of high-dose chemotherapy with stem cell or bone marrow transplantation.

Stage IV: Regardless of the size of the tumor in the breast, the definition of Stage IV means that the cancer has already spread to distant organs or to lymph nodes in the neck above the collar bone (supraclavicular lymph nodes).

Treatment Options for Stage IV: Systemic therapy is the primary treatment, using chemotherapy or hormonal therapy. Radiation and/or surgery may also be used to provide local control and to alleviate symptoms.

General Comments on Treatment Options by Stage: Women generally have more treatment options if the disease is diagnosed early. Treatment for DCIS depends on the extent of the tumor and its special features seen under the microscope. In Stages I and II, studies have shown that when patients are properly selected for breast conservation (i.e., lumpectomy), the survival results are the same as with mastectomy. Radiation therapy is not used after mastectomy except in the rare case that it was not possible to completely remove the tumor, or sometimes if there are four or more lymph nodes involved. Radiation is given in these circumstances to reduce the chance of skin or chest wall recurrence. To reduce the chance of recurrence elsewhere in the body, chemotherapy or hormone therapy may be given in Stages I and II. The type of adjuvant (additional) treatment selected depends on special features of the tumor, patient age, and menopausal status.

In Stage III, surgery and radiation are used to treat the larger tumor areas(s) in the breast and lymph nodes. Chemotherapy is necessary because the chances are high that distant spreading has occurred, but it is too small to find. Chemotherapy may be given before surgery or radiation to reduce the tumor size.

There are ongoing studies to evaluate the best sequence for treating breast cancer with chemotherapy, surgery, and radiation. Breast conservation therapy for Stage III patients is investigational at this point since the outcome is not yet known. Researchers are also investigating high-dose, stronger chemotherapy with or without bone marrow transplantation. With Stage IV breast cancer, the systemic treatment (chemotherapy) is the primary therapy. Surgery or radiation are used only for limited reasons. Each case is unique, and the cancer care team, consulting with the patient, should determine the best treatment.

[End of public domain materials.]

BREAST CANCER TREATMENTS— THEN AND NOW

It is important to know that significant progress has been made on the treatment of breast cancer. While researching the progress against breast cancer, I found an article by Marian Segal and Judith Levine Willis.[12] While the article does repeat some of the information we have discussed, it is a very important and informative overview of the progress made against this disease. In addition, I think women should be aware of the excellent publications provided by the Food and Drug Administration's Department of Health & Human Services. I have reproduced the article, "Progress Against Breast Cancer," as a public service and would encourage everyone, especially women, to read the other great articles in this special edition.

PROGRESS AGAINST BREAST CANCER
by Marian Segal and Judith Levine Willis

More than 20 years ago, Joyce Fine of Bethesda, Md., had a radical mastectomy to treat breast cancer. She didn't discuss her disease much with anyone then, except her husband.

In those days, Fine remembers, cancer was not talked about. "Everything was secretive then. Obituaries of people with cancer read that they died of 'a lingering illness'." Fine thinks that her father's mother may have had breast cancer, but she's not sure. The impression came from a single conversation she happened to overhear.

A New Attitude

Today people are not only open and truthful but often also activist about breast cancer. Along with strides in diagnosis and treatment have come long overdue changes in attitudes and awareness about the disease. Betty Ford, Nancy Reagan, Happy Rockefeller, Shirley Temple Black, Gloria Steinem, and many other public figures have come forward in recent years to tell about their experiences. But it's certainly not just because of the celebrities that breast cancer has captured the public's attention.

According to the American Cancer Society, breast cancer yearly strikes about 185,000 women and kills about 44,000. It is second only to lung cancer in cancer deaths in women. According to the National Cancer Institute (NCI) the disease strikes 1 in 8 American women (1 in 9 before age 85), so it's unusual not to know someone who has had breast cancer.

Yet progress is being made. In March 1997, NCI announced that for the first time since scientists began keeping cancer statistics in the 1930s, deaths from breast cancer had declined—by 6.3 percent from 1991 through 1995. This is part of an overall trend of decreasing cancer deaths.

Though the average lifetime risk of breast cancer for a woman is 1 in 8, a woman's risk of getting it in any given year is less than 1 in 100. A woman's risk rises continuously with age. According to NCI, on the average, a woman's risk of getting breast cancer is about: 1 in 19,600 by age 25; 1 in 2,500 by age 30; 1 in 200 by age 40; 1 in 50 by age 50; 1 in 24 by age

60; 1 in 14 by age 70; 1 in 10 by age 80; and by age 85, 1 in 9. Women whose mothers or sisters have had breast cancer have two to three times the usual risk of developing the disease. The risk is greatest if the relative developed breast cancer before menopause or if both breasts were involved. Nevertheless, hereditary breast cancer accounts for only 5 to 10 percent of breast cancer cases. As NCI researcher Susan Bates, M.D., says, the statement, "There's no breast cancer in my family" should provide a woman no security whatsoever.

Overall, breast cancer is more common in white women from North America and Northern Europe and in women of high socioeconomic status. However, African American women under 50 have a higher risk than white women of this age, while after age 50, the breast cancer risk of African American women is lower than for white women. Women of Eastern European (Ashkenazi) Jewish descent appear to be at higher risk than other groups due to genetic factors.

BRCA Genes

Alteration of a gene scientists named BRCA1 (for Breast Cancer 1) has been linked to the development of inherited breast cancer, as first reported in the Oct. 7, 1994, issue of the journal *Science*. The research was accomplished by the scientists of Myriad Genetics, Inc., the University of Utah, and the National Institutes of Health. This gene, located on chromosome 17, is one of several genes that, when normal, suppress the growth of tumors. BRCA1 has also been linked to familial ovarian cancer (see "Ovarian Cancer," page 111).

It has been estimated that women with a mutated BRCA1 gene may have a lifetime breast cancer risk of up to 85 percent (compared with about 12 percent for women in general). However, a report by Jeffrey P Struewing, M.D., and colleagues in the May 15, 1997, New England Journal of Medicine, indicates that the risk may be overestimated. In any case, it is important to note that not all women who have the BRCA1 alteration will develop breast cancer. The altered gene does not seem to increase breast cancer risk in men.

In the general U.S. population, this mutation occurs in 1 in 300 to 1 in 800 women. But it occurs in 1 of 10 Ashkenazi Jewish women. Two specific BRCA1 mutations have been identified in several families of Jewish Ashkenazi descent with a family history of breast cancer. The mutations are named 185delAG and 5382insC. In addition, NIH scientists reported in the Oct. 1, 1995, issue of *Nature Genetics* that mutation 185delAG had been found in blood samples of 1 percent (8 of 858) of Ashkenazi Jews whose family or personal cancer history was unknown. None of 815 blood samples of individuals not selected for ethnicity had this alteration.

NIH scientists are conducting follow-up studies of 3,000 to 5,000 people in the Washington, D.C., and Long Island, N.Y., Ashkenazi Jewish populations to see how the presence of this alteration correlates with cases of breast and ovarian cancer.

The alteration of a second gene, BRCA2, located on chromosome 13, is also linked to inherited breast cancer. This link was identified and first reported by researchers at Duke University and the United Kingdom's Institute for Cancer Research in the Dec. 21, 1996, issue of the journal *Nature*.

"BRCA1 seems to be responsible for about half of inherited breast cancers," said P. Andrew Futreal, M.D., one of the Duke University researchers. "Our findings strongly suggest that BRCA2 accounts for the remaining 50 percent."

Scientists have estimated that BRCA1 and BRCA2 mutations occur in more than 2 out of 100 Ashkenazi Jews. A study reported in the May 15, 1997, issue of the *New England Journal of Medicine* by Michael Krainer, M.D., and colleagues concludes that BRCA2 mutations may contribute to fewer cases of breast cancer in younger women (early onset) than do BRCA1 mutations. BRCA2 alteration appears to increase a woman's lifetime risk of ovarian cancer to about 10 percent. Families with the BRCA2 alteration also appear to have higher rates of male breast cancer, prostate cancer, and ocular melanoma (a type of eye cancer). A specific BRCA2 alteration, called 6174delT, has been identified in Ashkenazi Jewish families.

Most scientists in this field recommend that testing for these genes be limited to research in which subjects are members of families at high risk for either ovarian or breast cancer, and that genetic counseling and risk assessment—including the possibility of false-negative and false-positive results—be provided. A two-part report in the March 19 and March 26,

1997, issues of the *Journal of the American Medical Association* presents guidelines for doctors from the Cancer Genetics Studies Consortium, composed of government and nongovernment experts and organized by the National Human Genome Research Institute. The guidelines advise doctors to counsel patients to consider all ramifications of genetic tests before being tested. The guidelines also say that women who carry either of the BRCA genes should begin monthly breast self-exams when they are 18 to 21 years old and annual mammograms and breast exams by a health professional between the ages of 25 and 35.

Some women with a high genetic risk of breast cancer consider breast removal (when no cancer is present) as a way to prevent cancer. Such prophylactic surgery is controversial. A study reported by Deborah Schrag, M.D., and colleagues in the May 15, 1997 issue of the *New England Journal of Medicine* estimates that, on the average, 30-year-old women who carry BRCA1 or BRCA2 mutations gain about 3 to 5 years of life from such surgery. Gains in life expectancy decline with age and by the time a woman is 60 disappear. Women considering prophylactic surgery should be aware of all the issues involved, including the fact that such surgery does not completely eliminate the possibility of cancer.

Other Genetic and Risk Factors

The first tumor suppressor gene associated with breast cancer was reported in the Nov. 30, 1990, issue of Science by Stephen H. Friend, M.D., Ph.D., of the Massachusetts General Hospital Cancer Center. Certain alterations in a tumor suppressor gene called p53 lead to a rare syndrome involving increased susceptibility to a number of cancers, including early-onset breast cancer, certain childhood cancers, brain tumors, leukemias, and a tendency to develop multiple tumors. About 100 families around the world have been identified with this rare syndrome, named Li-Fraumeni for the two scientists who first described it in 1969. Follow-up of the four families originally identified 16 new cancer cases when only one would have been expected. Other relatively rare genetic mutations are also known to be associated with an increased risk of breast cancer. Certain types of benign (noncancerous) breast disease and radiation exposure are also established risk factors. Among postmenopausal women, obesity is associated with an increase in risk.

A link between radiation and breast cancer was established from studies of survivors of Hiroshima and Nagasaki and of women who had undergone radiation therapy or had repeated fluoroscopy, which was used many years ago to treat tuberculosis. The interval between exposure and disease development varies, but, according to Bates, the average is 20 years.

Women who begin menstruating before age 12, become menopausal after 50, delay childbearing until after 30, or who bear no children are also at higher risk. On the other hand, the risk is lower in women who have their first child before age 18 and in women who, because of surgical removal of the ovaries, become menopausal before age 35.

However, the American Cancer Society points out that about 25 percent of breast cancer cases occur among women with no major risk factors, so all women should consider themselves at risk.

Possible Risks

Reserpine (a drug for high blood pressure marketed as Rogroton, Ser-Ap-Es, Hydropres, and others), hair dye chemicals, cigarette smoking, alcohol consumption, dietary fat, birth control pills, and estrogen therapy have all been suggested as risk factors, but results from various studies have been contradictory, and their role in disease development remains controversial.

Some research has indicated that birth control pills might increase the risk of breast cancer, particularly in premenopausal women between the ages of 45 and 55, in women with a family history of breast cancer, or among young women who use them before the first pregnancy. One long-term study, however, reported that neither short-term nor long-term (more than 11 years) use appeared to increase risk, even in these groups of women. For now, the Food and Drug Administration requires that birth control pills carry a label indicating that the association between oral contraceptives and breast cancer is not clear.

Women who receive estrogen replacement therapy (ERT)

may also be at increased risk. ERT is recommended for some menopausal women to counteract hot flashes and sweating and to slow bone thinning (osteoporosis). ERT may also confer protection from cardiovascular disease. A study of 118,000 female nurses followed for 10 years found a "modest" increase in breast cancer risk in current users—more so with increasing age—but not in past users, even if therapy had lasted more than 10 years. The researchers, led by Graham Colditz, M.B., B.S. (British equivalent of M.D.), of Brigham and Women's Hospital in Boston, concluded that, "Though this increase in risk will be counterbalanced by the cardiovascular benefits, there is a need for caution in the use of estrogens."

It is not clear whether the addition of progestin to this regimen has any effect on breast cancer risk.

Another hormone scientists are investigating in relation to breast cancer is DES (diethylstilbestrol), prescribed a generation ago to prevent miscarriage and to prevent lactation after childbirth, and linked with vaginal cancer in daughters of mothers who took it while pregnant.

The possible relation of a high-fat diet and alcohol intake to breast cancer is also being investigated. The death rate from breast cancer is highest in countries, including the United States, in which the intake of fat and animal protein is high. For instance, Japanese women historically have a low risk for breast cancer, but that risk has been rising dramatically, concurrent with a "Westernization" of eating habits—that is, from a low-fat to a high-fat diet. Within Japan, the risk is 8.5 times higher for wealthier women, who eat meat daily, than among poorer women.

When large populations move from a low-incidence area to a high-incidence area and adopt the local lifestyle, they tend to take on the cancer risk patterns of their new homeland. Among immigrants from Asia to the United States, the incidence of breast cancer typically rises somewhat in the first generation, then continues to rise in subsequent generations until it approaches that of women born in the United States.

A study involving nearly 57,000 women published in the March 6, 1991, Journal of the National Cancer Institute, found an association between breast cancer and fat intake that, the author say, "appears unlikely to have arisen by chance," even though the link is not strong and two previous studies contradict their results. It could be that the issue is unclear because the difference in fat content between the lower fat and higher fat diets of the women studied may not be great enough to influence breast cancer development. Americans typically consume 40 percent of their calories in fat. A reduction to 30 percent may not be significant in reducing breast cancer risk.

To examine the question further, NIH's Women's Health Initiative includes a study of women aged 50 to 69 comparing those who greatly reduce their fat intake with those who don't to see how this difference in diet affects the incidence of breast cancer, colorectal cancer, heart disease, and overall mortality.

These risk factors may appear unrelated, but a possible common thread may be estrogen. Estrogen causes breast cells to grow, and there may be times in a woman's life when the breast is more susceptible to cancer-causing substances in the environment. A longer menstrual history, the additional estrogens from birth control pills or from ERT, or even a high-fat diet, alcohol intake, or just being overweight may increase the amount of estrogen in the bloodstream, increasing the amount available to the woman's breast tissue.

Anatomy of a Disease

The breast is a gland designed to produce milk. Milk ducts leading to the nipple originate from lobules inside 15 or 20 lobes arranged like spokes around a wheel. The spaces around and between the milk-producing lobes are filled with fat. About 90 percent of breast cancers arise from the milk ducts. When ductal carcinoma, as it is called, remains confined to the duct, it is called in situ, or intraductal, cancer. When the cells penetrate the walls of the duct and invade surrounding tissue, it is called invasive ductal cancer. About 5 percent of breast cancers are lobular carcinomas, which originate in the lobules.

Two atypical kinds of breast cancers are inflammatory breast carcinoma and Paget's disease. While most breast cancers are slow growing and painless, inflammatory breast cancer progresses very rapidly and is painful, with symptoms resembling an infection. The breast is warm and reddened, and the skin may appear pitted like an orange peel. In Paget's disease, the nipple becomes crusted; cancer cells grow upward along the ducts from a malignancy (cancer) deeper in the breast.

When an abnormality is detected in the breast by mammography (see "Mammography: A Lifesaving Step"), the doctor may recommend a biopsy. If a lump is found by palpation (feeling the mass), a biopsy is almost always necessary. Exceptions may be certain lumps found in women who have histories of lumpy or cystic breasts, and in some fluid-filled and solid tumors when imaging methods in addition to mammography are used. Any woman noticing a lump—especially if newly developed—should consult her doctor.

To help differentiate benign from cancerous tumors, in April 1996, FDA approved an additional use for a high definition ultrasound system as an adjunct to mammography and physician breast exam. The Ultramark 9 High Definition Imaging (HDI) Ultrasound System Level 3, originally cleared for marketing in 1991 for general-purpose imaging, including whether breast tumors are fluid-filled or solid, can now also be used to help assess whether a solid tumor is likely to be benign (fluid-filled tumors in younger women are almost always benign). Before this approval, solid tumors had to be biopsied to ensure correct diagnosis. The HDI system is approved for use in diagnosing tumors that are at least 1 centimeter (about three-eighths of an inch) in diameter.

The biopsy usually involves surgical removal of all or part of the lump or suspicious area, allowing a pathologist to examine the tissue and determine with certainty whether or not the lesion is cancerous. Some biopsies are done by fine needle aspiration, using a local anesthetic. The doctor inserts a needle into the lump and tries to withdraw fluid. If it is a cyst, it will collapse when the fluid is removed. If it is solid, the doctor may remove some cells with the needle to send to the laboratory for analysis. About 80 percent of palpable lumps are benign (not cancerous).

Biopsy does not always require hospitalization. It can be done as an outpatient procedure. Until the late 1970s, it was standard procedure for the patient having a biopsy to sign a consent form permitting the surgeon to remove the breast at the same time if the tumor was found to be cancerous. The common practice nowadays is to do a biopsy first and then schedule surgery, if necessary, within the next few weeks. Some women may still choose the one-step procedure that was routine when Joyce Fine had her mastectomy.

The interval with the two-step procedure, however, allows the woman time to find out about and choose among her treatment options, get a second opinion, and prepare for her hospital stay. The brief delay in treatment does not reduce the chances for a successful outcome. Some states have passed laws requiring that women be told a two-step procedure is their legal right and, in some cases, that they be given specific information about their options.

Progress in Therapy

The treatment options women have today were not available to Joyce Fine when she had her mastectomy—a Halsted radical. This entailed removing the entire breast, underlying chest muscles, all the axillary (underarm) lymph nodes, and some additional fat and muscle. Fine's surgeon did not discuss with her possible treatment alternatives. The Halsted radical was the standard treatment for breast cancer in 1972.

"There was no discussion," Fine recalls. "He convinced me I had to have the tumor out as soon as possible and that I should sign a release that if they find at biopsy that it's cancerous, they should remove it right away."

The surgeon acknowledged that Fine could have a two-step procedure. "But he said that if I go that way, it would metastasize [spread] and I couldn't be put under anesthesia again soon," she says. "It would be a waiting period of a couple of weeks, and I was so frightened I said I'd do it in one procedure. He made me feel as though if I didn't, I might be dead in two weeks."

And so, like so many women with breast cancer then, Fine went into surgery not knowing if she would leave the hospital physically the same as she entered, or minus one breast as the result of extensive, disfiguring surgery.

"Beginning in the 1940s, studies were suggesting that so much surgery was not necessary," said NCI's Bates. "In Europe, by 1971, smaller operations were accepted, but in the

United States, change was slow in coming. Surgeons were reluctant to abandon the Halsted radical mastectomy for fear of giving inadequate treatment."

Treating Early-Stage Disease

Both the Halstad surgery and the process Fine experienced now belong to medical history. It is generally agreed that radical surgery is not helpful if the cancer has spread, and not necessary if the cancer has not spread. Surgical treatment now emphasizes breast conservation—preserving the breast when possible. Lumpectomy (also called segmental mastectomy or tylectomy), in which only the tumor and a margin of surrounding tissue is removed, is now common treatment for breast cancer. This procedure is light years away from the Halsted radical, both in its physical and psychological effects.

Radical mastectomy was based on the rationale that breast cancer started with a tumor in the breast and, over time, spread in an orderly fashion to the lymph glands under the arms and then, through the lymph and blood, to other parts of the body—usually the lungs, liver, bone, or brain. Halsted's procedure was designed to remove the avenues of possible spread.

By the late 1970s, experts had determined that the Halsted radical mastectomy was not necessary. This conclusion was based on research that changed the concept of how breast cancer progresses. It is now understood that very early in the disease (although exactly how early is not known), breast cancer cells travel through the blood and lymph to other parts of the body. In this process, called micrometastasis, the cancer is so small it can't even be detected with a microscope. In other cases, depending on the biology of the cancer cells, the cancer may remain in the breast without spreading until later in the course of the disease.

Treatment now emphasizes removing the tumor while sparing the breast. By examining tissue taken during surgery, doctors can see if tumors may have spread. Patients with such tumors then can receive additional therapy, which may include radiation, chemotherapy (drugs that kill cancer cells), hormone therapy, or a combination.

As new approaches to surgical and medical treatment have been tried, each method has had its supporters and dissenters. In 1957, NCI organized the National Surgical Adjuvant Breast Project to create a pool of data gathered from research on breast cancer treatments. In the late 1970s, scientists reviewed study results and determined that simple, or total, mastectomy, in which only the breast was removed, was as effective as the Halsted radical.

Then, in 1990, at an NIH consensus development conference on treatment of early-stage breast cancer, a panel of experts agreed that still less-extensive surgery, lumpectomy, gave the same results if radiation followed surgery to kill any remaining cancer cells. The lymph nodes are also removed for examination during this procedure.

The panel concluded that breast conservation treatment is not only appropriate for most women with early-stage disease but also "is preferable because it provides survival equivalent to total mastectomy and also preserves the breast. Total mastectomy remains an appropriate primary therapy when breast conservation is not indicated or selected."

Women who have multicentric breast cancer (cancers that develop at several locations within a single breast), or whose tumors are large relative to breast size and therefore would not have a good cosmetic result, are among those who may not be candidates for breast conservation.

No single procedure can be recommended as ideal for all patients. Women and their surgeons must base their decisions on the patient's medical status and her particular concerns. Her choice may be influenced by emotional considerations, finances, access to care, body image, and personal beliefs.

Following either mastectomy or lumpectomy with radiation, additional (adjuvant) therapy is given to most women whose cancer has spread to the lymph nodes. This may be chemotherapy or hormone therapy, or both. A current controversy in treatment concerns whether or not to treat node-negative breast cancer patients (patients in whom the disease has not spread to the lymph nodes) with adjuvant therapy, since these additional treatments to improve the outcome can also have side effects. Seven of 10 node-negative women will never have a recurrence of disease. Of the remaining three, standard adjuvant therapy will prevent recurrence in one.

Unfortunately, there is no way yet to predict which three

will have a recurrence, nor which one of those will be helped by adjuvant treatment. The dilemma, says Bates, is, "Do we treat 10 to help one, and potentially three, if our treatments can improve?"

Many drugs have been tried alone and in combination to find the best treatment. Cancer drugs can have serious side effects. They are designed to kill cancer cells, but they also affect other rapidly growing cells, such as bloodforming cells in the bone marrow and those that line the digestive tract. As a result, they may lower resistance to infection, sap energy, and cause bruising or bleeding, nausea, vomiting, mouth sores, loss of appetite, hair loss, reduced heart function, and other side effects. Premenopausal women may also experience hot flashes, vaginal dryness, painful intercourse, and irregular menstrual periods.

Side effects of chemotherapy vary with each patient, according to the treatment given and the individual's reaction. Severe vomiting can be a problem. However, FDA has approved drugs such as Zofran (ondansetron hydrochloride) to treat the nausea and vomiting associated with chemotherapy. Marinol (oral marijuana derivative) has also been effective in selected cases.

Tamoxifen

An oral drug called tamoxifen (marketed as Nolvadex) is most often given to women whose cancer cells are estrogen-receptor positive— that is, their growth is likely to be encouraged by estrogen. Tamoxifen interferes with the activity of estrogen, thus keeping the cells from getting the hormones they need to grow. Originally approved by FDA in 1977 for patients with advanced breast cancer and subsequently for patients with less severe disease, tamoxifen was also approved for use in node-negative patients in June 1990.

Tamoxifen slows or stops the growth of cancer cells already present in the body and helps prevent recurrence and development of cancer in the other breast. Though the drug counters the effects of estrogen in breast tissue, it acts like estrogen in other parts of the body, so that women taking the drug may receive benefits similar to that of hormone replacement therapy, such as lowering of blood cholesterol and slowing of bone loss after menopause.

Possible adverse effects include a risk of blood clots similar to birth control pills, and an elevated risk of uterine cancer. More common but less serious side effects include hot flashes, nausea and vomiting. Patients may also experience visual changes and develop cataracts.

FDA has approved a blood test to help determine whether breast cancer has recurred. Called the Truquant BR Radioimmunoassy Kit, it measures an antigen found in the blood of patients with breast cancer, as well as other types of cancer. Test results can be analyzed within a few hours in a hospital lab. However, because there can be false-positive and false-negative results, it is not intended as the sole basis for detection of cancer recurrence. This diagnosis can only be made after the test results are verified by other diagnostic procedures.

Treating Advanced Disease

Breast cancer that has advanced to Stage III or IV (see accompanying article, "Determining Therapy") requires chemotherapy or hormone therapy, or both, to treat its spread. Treatment may also include surgery or radiation therapy, or both, to control the breast tumor. Hormone therapy may be accomplished with drugs such as tamoxifen or, in premenopausal women, by removing the hormone-producing ovaries. Women whose cancer has spread beyond the breast to other parts of the body usually have less extensive breast surgery, but receive hormonal therapy or more aggressive chemotherapy directed to treating both local and metastatic disease. If necessary, radiation may be used for local control.

Most tumors eventually become resistant to anticancer drugs and continue to grow. New treatments under study for patients with advanced breast cancer involve removing some of the patient's bone marrow and administering chemotherapy at very high doses to overcome drug resistance. This is followed by reinfusing the bone marrow to prevent life-threatening drug toxicity. This therapy is also being tried in patients at high risk of disease recurrence.

Other means of reversing drug resistance with various agents are under study. One such agent, verapamil (approved for treating high blood pressure), has been shown in laboratory studies to block a cell surface protein that pumps chemo-

therapy drugs out of a cell, thereby making it drug resistant.
Fortunately, most breast cancers are now detected at the earlier, more treatable stages. According to NCI, about 59 percent of women diagnosed with breast cancer in 1986-1992 had small, localized tumors, and about 32 percent had cancer that was regionally confined. According to the American Cancer Society, the five-year survival rate for localized breast cancer has risen from 78 percent in the 1940s to about 96 percent today. However, some breast cancers, even though localized, will recur after five years. The overall 10-year survival rate is 65 percent, and after 15 years it is 56 percent.

Though much progress has been made, much remains to be done. For example, though death rates have begun to fall for the general population, in certain groups, such as African Americans, they are not decreasing as rapidly as in the general population. This points out the need for continued education about diagnosis and treatment. Too, knowledge about the role of heredity and the environment in this disease is still unfolding.

And research continues. Some areas of investigation include alternate methods of diagnosis, such as 3-dimensional x-rays and other forms of imaging, simpler biopsy procedures, and more effective drugs and combinations of drugs.

It is important to remember that every woman should consider herself at risk for breast cancer. A woman's best tool in fighting this disease is knowledge—of her body (through examination by a health professional, mammography, and breast self-exam), of her family history, and of other risk factors. Such knowledge can go far to ensure early diagnosis and prompt treatment if she should be among the 12 percent of American women stricken with breast cancer during their lives.

[Marian Segal is a member of FDA's public affairs staff Judith Levine Willis is editor of this special issue.]

Determining Therapy

Treatment is based on the extent of the disease and the biology of the specific tumor. Evaluation of these factors guides the approach of surgery and, if needed, adjuvant therapy. In addition, a woman's age and menopausal status are significant. Breast cancer tends to be more aggressive in younger, premenopausal women.

First, based on tumor size and degree of cancer spread, the disease is classified into one of the following stages:

- **Carcinoma *in situ*:** Very early breast cancer that has not invaded nearby tissues.
- **Stage I:** Localized tumor no larger than 2 centimeters (cm) (about 1 inch).
- **Stage II:** Tumor no larger than 2 cm, but the cancer has spread to the underarm lymph nodes, or tumor between 2 and 5 cm (about 2 inches) and cancer may not have spread to the lymph nodes, or tumor bigger than 5 cm, but cancer has not spread to the lymph nodes.
- **Stage III:** Tumor larger than 5 cm and cancer has spread to underarm lymph nodes, or tumor smaller than 5 cm and the underarm lymph nodes have grown into each other or into other tissues, or the tumor has spread to tissues near the breast (such as the chest muscles and ribs) or to lymph nodes near the collarbone, or it is inflammatory breast cancer.
- **Stage IV:** The cancer has spread to other organs of the body, usually the lungs, liver, bone, or brain.

Carcinoma *in situ* has a cure rate approaching 100 percent with surgery alone. Tumors of 1 cm or less also carry a particularly good prognosis—less than 10 percent recurrence in 10 years. In general, the risk of recurrence rises with increasing tumor size and lymph node involvement.

Breast tumor tissue can be examined for important "markers" that give clues to the aggressiveness of the disease and can, therefore, help guide therapy. Some of these Tumor sizes in centimeters markers are:

- **Estrogen and progesterone receptors.** Patients whose cancer cells have proteins (receptors) to which these hormones bind have a better prognosis because the cells can be treated with hormone therapy.
- **Histologic type.** Breast cancers vary in their cell type. For example, invasive ductal cancers can sometimes be categorized into further subtypes, such a mucinous, tubular and medullary. Lobular cancers are another cell type. The various types have different rates of growth and spread.
- **DNA studies.** The degree of disruption of DNA in the cell nucleus correlates with the disease aggressiveness. The

more disarrayed the DNA, the greater the risk of relapse. Also, cells that divide more rapidly carry a poorer prognosis.
• **HER-2 oncogene.** This gene is sometimes found in tumors of patients whose cancer has spread. Detected early, it might predict spread and identify patients who would benefit from more aggressive treatment.
• **Cathepsin D.** High levels of this protein are associated with a poorer prognosis. Secreted by the cancer cells, cathepsin D may aid their spread to other parts of the body.

Mammography: A Lifesaving Step

Mammography can be lifesaving. It is widely agreed that women 50 and over should have a mammogram yearly. Widespread mammography screening programs for women in this age group can reduce breast cancer death rates by 30 percent, according to a seven major randomized controlled clinical trials. This is especially important for older women, since the incidence of breast cancer increases dramatically with age.

Mammography is the best method available for detecting tumors in their early stages. It help can detect 85 to 90 percent of breast cancers in women over 50 and can discover a tumor up to two years before a doctor or patient would otherwise know it was there.

For women aged 40 to 49, the following recommendations had recently been made when this special issue went to press in the spring of 1997:

• National Institutes of Health independent consensus panel: No single recommendation for screening of all women in this age group. After weighing the benefits and risks with her doctor, each woman should decide whether to have yearly mammograms before age 50.

• National Cancer Institute: Mammography screening every one to two years.

• American Cancer Society: Mammography screening once a year.

The differences in recommendations stem from differences in interpretations of the studies. According to the NIH panel experts, studies do not show that yearly mammographic screening has clear benefits for women in their 40s when relative risks for women in this age group are taken into account.

These risks include a higher percentage of false-positive readings than for older women (30 percent of women aged 40 to 49 who have mammograms are told an abnormality exists when none does). These false-positive readings can result in unnecessary tests and surgery. When women in this age group undergo biopsies after a positive mammogram, half as many cancers are found as among women aged 50 to 59. Of every eight biopsies in the 40-to-49-year-old age group, one invasive and one in situ breast cancer is found. In addition, the rate of false-negative readings is high in this group: In women 40 to 49 years old, mammography misses 25 percent of invasive breast cancer compared with 10 percent in older women.

Further, the NIH panel said that studies showed no differences in breast cancer death rates within seven years between women in their 40s who had had mammography and those who had not.

Nevertheless, there may be compelling reasons for yearly mammograms for women in their 40s. For example, although the studies individually did not show a clear-cut benefit, when data from all the studies were pooled, they showed about a 17 percent reduction in deaths among women who had had mammograms. In addition, most of the studies included only white women. Although the incidence of breast cancer is about the same for white and African American women, in this age group, African American women have a 50 percent higher breast cancer death rate than white women.

It is important to note that all age-related screening recommendations apply to women who have no symptoms of breast cancer and who are not at increased risk for the disease. Any woman, regardless of age, should see her doctor immediately if she has symptoms, such as a lump, nipple discharge, or other change in the breast. And, for women who have no symptoms but may be at higher risk because of genetic or family history, or late childbearing, for example, a physician may recommend earlier and more frequent mammograms.

It is important that mammography be of the highest possible quality. Mammography can fail to do its job due to poor technique in taking, processing or reading the films; inadequate record keeping and reporting of results; and lack of effective quality controls.

The concern that facilities varied in the quality of mammograms performed and the desire for high-quality mammography in all facilities resulted in Congress passing the Mammography Quality Standards Act (MQSA) in 1992.

FDA has the responsibility for implementing and enforcing the MQSA. In December 1993, the agency set forth standards that mammography professionals and facilities would have to meet by Oct. 1, 1994, or stop doing mammography. When this special issue went to press, FDA was expected to publish final rules later in 1997.

In accordance with the law, all mammography facilities must be certified by FDA-approved accreditation bodies. To be certified, a facility must meet quality standards for x-ray images, equipment and personnel and must be inspected annually. By early 1997, all U.S. facilities had been inspected at least once, and two-thirds had had their second annual inspection. There are now about 10,060 certified mammography facilities in the United States.

When selecting a facility, women should find out if it is certified by FDA. If a facility is certified by FDA, Medicare will provide reimbursement for qualified patients. Women who have breast implants should ask if the facility uses special techniques designed for women with implants.

FDA has posted a list of facilities it has certified, divided by state, at http://www.fda.gov/cdrh/faclist.html on the agency's World Wide Web site.

Breast Self-Examination (BSE)

Breast self-examination should be done once a month so you become familiar with the usual appearance and feel of your breasts. Familiarity makes it easier to notice any changes in the breast from one month to another. Early discovery of a change from what is "normal" is the main idea behind BSE. If you menstruate, the best time to do BSE is two or three days after your period ends, when your breasts are least likely to be tender or swollen. If you no longer menstruate, pick a day, such as the first day of the month, to remind yourself it is time to do BSE.

1. Stand before a mirror. Inspect both breasts for anything

unusual, such as any discharge from the nipples, puckering, dimpling, or scaling of the skin.

The next two steps are designed to emphasize any change in the shape or contour of your breasts. As you do them, you should be able to feel your chest muscles tighten.

2. Watching closely in the mirror, clasp hands behind your head and press hands forward.

3. Next, press hands firmly on hips and bow slightly toward the mirror as you pull your shoulders and elbows forward.

Some women do the next part of the exam in the shower. Fingers glide over soapy skin, making it easy to concentrate on the texture underneath.

4. Raise your left arm. Use three or four fingers of your right hand to explore your left breast firmly, carefully and thoroughly. Beginning at the outer edge, press the flat part of your fingers in small circles, moving the circles slowly around the breast. Gradually work toward the nipple. Be sure to cover the entire breast. Pay special attention to the area between the breast and the armpit, including the armpit itself. Feel for any unusual lump or mass under the skin.

5. Gently squeeze the nipple and look for a discharge. Repeat the exam on your right breast. (If you have any discharge during the month—whether or not it is during BSE—see your doctor.)

6. Steps 4 and 5 should be repeated lying down. Lie flat on your back, left arm over your head and a pillow or folded towel under your left shoulder. This position flattens the breast and makes it easier to examine. Use the same circular motion described earlier. Repeat on your right breast.

Reconstruction Options

Breast reconstruction after mastectomy used to be very complex, and the results were often disappointing. So, as recently as a generation ago, few women chose to have it done and many were not aware it was a possibility. In the last quarter of this century, however, advances in plastic surgery have made breast reconstruction easier, more successful, and more popular.

Still, not every woman who has had a mastectomy chooses

reconstruction. Some women decide against it because they don't want to have more surgery or they feel the risks outweigh the benefits or for other reasons. Many women prefer to wear breast forms (prostheses).

For women who desire reconstruction, however, there are few limitations. Even women who have had radical surgery or whose skin has been grafted, damaged by radiation therapy, or is otherwise thin or tight can have successful reconstructive surgery.

Although some women have breast reconstruction during the same surgery as their mastectomy, many surgeons recommend waiting three to six months. This allows time to complete radiation or chemotherapy and for the mastectomy incision to heal.

Three major types of breast reconstruction are available.

Implant Placement

There are two types of breast implants currently available for reconstruction patients. One is filled with saline (salt water), the other with silicone gel. Both types have a silicone envelope. Since April 1992, the use of silicone gel-filled implants has been limited to women participating in clinical trials designed to evaluate the risks and benefits of the devices. Saline implants are available without restriction. (See "A Status Report on Breast Implant Safety," page 100.) The most common problem associated with both saline and gel-filled breast implants is capsular contracture. This occurs when scar tissue shrinks around the implant, making it feel hard and sometimes misshaping it. Other known health risks include incorrect mammography results, implant rupture, and change in breast sensation, which may be temporary or permanent. In addition, silicone gel can escape from gel-filled implants because of rupture. Small quantities of silicone also "bleed" from intact implants.

Like the silicone gel-filled devices, saline implants have a silicone rubber envelope and may not be entirely without risk. In addition, with leakage or rupture, saline implants deflate and usually must be replaced. Women considering implants need to be aware that repeat surgeries may be required.

Latissimus Dorsi

"Latissimus dorsi" reconstruction gets its name from the broad flat back muscle that the surgeon moves to the chest to take the place of muscles that have been removed during the mastectomy. The surgeon also transfers skin and other tissue from the patient's back to the mastectomy site. An implant is then placed under the new muscle, and drains may be inserted temporarily. This operation takes longer and requires longer hospitalization than simple implant placement. It leaves a scar on the back in addition to the mastectomy scar on the chest.

Rectus Abdominus

In this procedure, the surgeon transfers one of two abdominal muscles to the breast area with skin and fat from the abdomen. The surgeon shapes this flap of muscle, skin and fat into the contour of a breast. If there is enough abdominal tissue available, no implant is needed. This procedure leaves a horizontal scar across the lower abdomen in addition to the mastectomy scar.

Nipple and Areola Construction

Breast reconstruction fashions the shape of the breast but does not always include a reconstructed nipple and areola (the dark skin around the nipple). Some women, who wish primarily to improve their appearance in clothing, choose not to have the additional one-to two-hour operation to reconstruct the nipple and areola. During this operation, the areola is usually fabricated from skin on the upper thigh or from behind the ear, and the nipple is created either from tissue from the newly created breast mound or from the other nipple. If the reconstructed areola is not dark enough, ultraviolet light can be used to darken the skin.

Although breast reconstruction offers a more normal appearance both in and out of clothes, women should be aware that if there are scars from these operations they are permanent and that reconstruction does not restore lost sensation.

For More Information

Here are the phone numbers and World Wide Web addresses of some of the many sources of breast cancer information:

General Information
National Cancer Institute's Cancer Information Service (CIS) (1-800) 4-CANCER (1-800-422-6237)
http://icisun.nci.nih.gov/occdocs/cis/cis.html

NCI's CancerNet
http://wwwicic.nci.nih.gov/

National Alliance of Breast Cancer Organizations (NABCO) (1-800) 719-9154 http:l/www. nabco.org/

The American Cancer Society
(1-800) ACS-2345 (1-800-227-2345)
http://www. cancer. org/bcn. html

Y-ME National Breast Cancer Organization
(1-800) 221-2141
http://www.y-me.org/index.html

OncoLink
http://www.oncolink.upenn. edu/disease/ breast/

Breast Cancer Information Center
http://feminist.org/other/bc/behome.html

EduCare, Inc.
http://www. cancerhelp com/ed/

Mammography
List of FDA-certified mammography facilities
http://www.fda.gov/ cdrh/faclist.html

American College of Radiology
http://www. acr. org/

[End of article.]

DEFINITIONS OF BREAST CANCER TERMS

Definitions of Treatment

Local Therapy: Local therapy typically involves a variety of surgical procedures to remove the tumor and varying amounts of surrounding tissue and to take samples of axillary lymph nodes under the arm. Local therapy may also include radiation treatments.

Fine-Needle Aspiration Biopsy (FNAB)—FNAB uses a thin needle, about the size of a needle used for blood tests or for immunizations. The needle can be guided into the area of the breast abnormality while the doctor is feeling or palpating a lump. It may even be guided into an abnormality too small to feel by using breast ultrasound examination or a mammographically-guided stereotactic biopsy apparatus.

Stereotactic biopsy is an accurate procedure in which an x-ray-guided needle takes a sample of a suspicious area that is discovered on a mammogram, but that is too small to be felt by either the patient or her doctor. This procedure is often used to biopsy calcifications (calcium deposits). A computer precisely controls the placement of the needle.

Applying suction to the needle (aspiration) during FNAB may yield fluid. Clear fluid usually indicates a benign cyst, while bloody or cloudy fluid may be present in benign cysts or cancers. FNAB of solid (not fluid-filled) abnormalities yields small tissue fragments. Microscopic examination of FNAB samples can determine whether most breast abnormalities are benign or cancerous. In some cases, a clear answer is not obtained by FNAB and another type of biopsy is needed.

Core biopsy—The needle used in core biopsies is larger than that used in FNAB. It removes a small cylinder of tissue from a breast abnormality. The biopsy is done with local anesthesia in the doctor's office. As with FNAB, a core biopsy can sample abnormalities felt by the doctor as well as smaller ones localized by ultrasound or stereotactic methods.

Nipple discharge procedures—If there is a nipple discharge, some of the fluid may be collected. The fluid is then examined under a microscope to determine if any cancer cells are present. A special x-ray may also be performed after injecting x-ray contrast material into the duct or ducts from which the spontaneous discharge is coming.

Surgical biopsy—Surgical removal of all, or a portion, of the lump for microscopic analysis may be required in some cases.

Today, most health professionals prefer a **two-step biopsy**. In this method, the biopsy usually can be done in the doctor's office or hospital outpatient department under a non-general anesthesia with intravenous sedation or local anesthesia where the woman is awake during the procedure. If the diagnosis is cancer, there is time to learn about it, discuss all treatment options with the cancer care team, friends, and family. The short delay until treatment does no harm. Of course, a diagnosis made by needle biopsy counts as the first step of a two-step procedure.

In earlier years, the only choice a woman had was a **one-step biopsy**. With this approach, she was given general anesthesia and was asleep during the entire process. A biopsy was performed and the tissue sample was frozen. The frozen sample was examined in the pathology laboratory under a microscope. If cancer cells were present, the surgeon immediately proceeded with treatment, such as mastectomy which the patient had previously approved. She did not know until she woke up whether the lump was cancerous and whether surgery was performed. This approach is rarely recommended.

Estrogen/Progesterone Receptors—Receptors are part of the molecular structure of a cell, functioning as a "welcome mat" for certain substances that circulate in the blood. Certain tumor cells have hormone receptors which will recognize estrogen and progesterone. These two substances play an important role in the development, treatment, and prognosis of certain tumors. An important step in evaluating a person with early breast cancer is to test for the presence of these receptors. This is done on a portion of the cancerous tissue to be removed at the time of biopsy or initial surgical treatment. Knowledge about your receptors provides important information relating to future hormone therapy which can affect the outlook, or prognosis, of a woman's breast cancer.

Breast Conservation

Lumpectomy involves the removal of only the lump and a

rim of normal tissue. Some of the underarm lymph nodes may be removed to see if the cancer has spread. Lumpectomy is almost always followed by several weeks of radiation therapy.

Partial or segmental mastectomy or quadrantectomy results in removal of up to one-quarter or more of the breast, depending on the findings. Axillary lymph nodes under the arm may also be removed. Radiation therapy is usually given following surgery. More breast tissue is lost in this method than in a lumpectomy.

Side effects of lumpectomy or partial mastectomy—There may be swelling, tenderness, and hardness in the surgical site for some time after the operation.

Simple or total mastectomy involves the removal of the entire breast.

Modified radical mastectomy involves the removal of the entire breast and axillary lymph nodes.

Radical mastectomy is the very extensive removal of the entire breast, axillary lymph nodes, and the chest wall muscles under the breast. This surgery was once very common, but because of its disfigurement and side effects, is now rarely done.

Side effects of mastectomy: Side effects include wound infection, hematoma (accumulation of blood in the wound), and seroma (accumulation of clear fluid in the wound). There may be limitations in arm and shoulder movement. A woman's cancer care team can help with these side effects, as well as the psychological and emotional consequences of mastectomy. Also, the American Cancer Society has programs which can help women facing breast cancer learn more about treatments and cope with treatment side effects.

Side effects of removal of lymph nodes: An uncommon (about 10-12%) side effect is lymphedema, swelling of the arm. There are measures to help prevent or reduce the effects of lymphedema. Women experiencing swelling, tightness or pain in the arm should be sure to tell the nurse or doctor promptly. Numbness of the upper inner arm skin is a common side effect.

Reconstructive surgery and breast implant surgery are not procedures to treat cancer, but to restore normal appearance after the mastectomy. If you expect that you will have a mastectomy and require reconstruction, it's important to consult **before** the operation with a plastic surgeon who is expert in breast reconstruction. Decisions about the type of reconstruction and when it will be done depend on your unique circumstances. You may find it helpful to talk with a woman who has had the type of reconstruction you are considering. The American Cancer Society's Reach to Recovery volunteers can assist you.

Systemic Therapy is given through the bloodstream. Surgery is an example of local treatment, while chemotherapy and hormonal therapy are systemic therapies. Systemic therapy is also called **adjuvant therapy** when it is given to patients with no cancer detectable after surgery. While doctors once believed that the metastasis of breast cancer could be controlled with extensive surgery at the primary site, this theory has been reconsidered. It is now believed that cancer cells may break away from the primary tumor and begin to spread through the bloodstream even in the early stages of the disease. These cells can't be felt by physical examination or seen on x-rays or other imaging methods, and they cause no symptoms. But they can establish new tumors in other organs or the bones. The goal of adjuvant therapy is to kill these hidden cells and tumors by using therapy that is systemic, which means that it reaches cancer cells throughout the body. Not every patient needs adjuvant therapy, especially if the cancer has been diagnosed very early, or if it is a slow-growing or very small tumor, or if the diagnosis is DCIS (ductal carcinoma in situ) or LCIS (lobular carcinoma in situ), considered by many researchers to be a precancerous condition rather than an actual cancer.

Chemotherapy is treatment with powerful anticancer drugs that may be given by injection into a blood vessel, and occasionally, by mouth. The drugs travel throughout the body in the bloodstream. Frequently, a combination of anticancer drugs is used because that has proven more effective than relying on a single drug. Chemotherapy is given in cycles, each followed by time for recovery. Then another period of treatment is followed by a recovery period, and so on. The total course of chemotherapy is often about six months, usually ranging from four to nine months. Chemotherapy can reduce the risk of cancer recurrence significantly. The exact risk of recurrence and benefit of chemotherapy depends on your specific situation.

The **side effects of chemotherapy** depend on the type of drugs, the amount taken, and the length of treatment. They include:
- Nausea and vomiting (New medications now can be given with the chemotherapy drugs to prevent these unpleasant side effects.)
- Loss or increase of appetite
- Temporary loss of hair (alopecia)
- Mouth or vaginal sores
- Increased chance of infections, bleeding, or anemia (low red blood cells)
- Fatigue
- Changes in the menstrual cycle
- Infertility (inability to become pregnant)

Chemotherapy during pregnancy: If a woman with breast cancer is pregnant or considering getting pregnant, she should tell her doctors before making decisions about her treatment. Some drugs used in chemotherapy are harmful to a fetus.

Acute myeloid leukemia (AML): A few of the anticancer drugs may rarely cause this life-threatening cancer of white blood cells. Most of the offending drugs are known and these are generally not used in current therapy of breast cancer. The rare chance that any of these drugs will cause leukemia is offset by their known positive effects against breast cancer.

Most of these side effects of chemotherapy (except infertility) stop when the treatment is over. There are remedies for many of the side effects. A woman should tell her cancer care team about any side effects she experiences.

Radiotherapy is radiation treatment which is given to destroy breast cancer cells. This treatment may be used to reduce the size of a tumor before surgery or to destroy cancer cells remaining after surgery.

Side effects—Many women complain of fatigue. If fatigue is a problem, the woman should discuss it with her cancer care team. There may be things she can do to obtain relief. Radiation may also cause some swelling and heaviness in the breast. This usually goes away in six to 12 months. The skin in the treated area may look and feel sunburned. This gradually fades to a tanned look, again returning to a normal appearance in six to 12 months. In some women, the breast becomes smaller and firmer. If a woman with breast cancer is pregnant or considering getting pregnant, she should tell her doctors before making decisions about her treatment. Radiotherapy is usually avoided during pregnancy because it can be harmful to a fetus.

Hormone Therapy can counter the growth of some breast cancer cells which can be encouraged by the female hormone, estrogen. The drug used most often is **tamoxifen** (brand named Nolvadex). Taken daily in pill form, tamoxifen enters the bloodstream and travels throughout the body. This means that the medicine affects all cells, not just tumor cells. Women taking tamoxifen should avoid getting pregnant because tamoxifen can damage the cells of a fetus. If a woman is already pregnant, she should tell her doctor before they discuss treatment decisions. Tamoxifen treatment lasts at least two years and often five years. Studies indicate the drug can reduce recurrence of breast cancer by 25% to 35%.

Side Effects of Tamoxifen—Some studies have shown a slightly increased occurrence of endometrial cancer (a cancer of the lining of the uterus) in a small number of women taking tamoxifen, with the risk increasing if the drug is taken for more than five years. Other effects may include weight gain, hot flashes, mood swings, and other symptoms. Any such side effects should be reported to the cancer care team. There may be ways to get relief from these side effects.

There are various other less common ways to manipulate hormones to reduce growth of breast cancer cells.

Progestins, estrogens, androgens—Adding progestins, estrogens and androgens may be considered after other hormone treatments have been tried. Side effects depend on the drugs used, but the most common is fluid retention. Androgens (male hormones) cause masculine characteristics to occur (more body hair, deeper voice, **and other symptoms**).

Oophorectomy—This is surgery to remove the ovaries. In women who have not gone through menopause, or the change of life, this surgery eliminates the body's main source of estrogen which promotes growth of some breast tumors.

Autologous Stem Cell and Bone Marrow Transplantation—The availability of stem cells, either from a woman's own bone marrow or her blood, makes it possible to use very high doses of chemotherapy or radiation to kill cancer cells. These powerful treatments also kill healthy cells, especially the white blood cells that fight infections. While the white blood cell count is low in an intensively treated patient, the patient is vulnerable to infections and death. To "rescue" the patient, stem cells from either the peripheral blood or bone marrow, are placed in the body. They soon establish themselves and restore the body's ability to fight infection. "Growth factors" may be added to the cells to boost the process of stem cell growth.

To perform either peripheral blood stem cell (PBSC) transplants or bone marrow transplants, it is necessary to collect and store the stem cells. These cells help create other cells. For a bone marrow transplant, cells are drawn from the hip bone. For a PBSC transplant, peripheral blood, which is the blood in general circulation throughout the body, is drawn from a vein. Then the blood is circulated through a high-speed cell separator. The stem cells are collected and stored for later use, and the plasma and red blood cells are returned to the patient.

Transplantation of peripheral blood stem cells offers advantages over the traditional bone marrow transplantation. It can be used even when cancer cells have spread to the bone marrow. In most cases, it can be done on an outpatient basis and does not require general anesthesia.

What's New in Breast Cancer Research and Treatment?

New areas currently under investigation include:

Monoclonal antibodies—These antibodies can be engineered to carry drugs or radiation directly to the tumor and may offer a way to treat micrometastases.

Metastasis- Metastasis is a complicated process of cells breaking away from the primary tumor, entering the blood supply, and relocating in other organs. Currently, researchers are working to define the steps in the breakdown of tissues that must occur before the tumor migrates to other locations, and grows larger.

Angiogenesis—Growth of cancers often depends on their ability to promote growth of blood vessels to nourish the cancer cells. Analysis of angiogenesis in breast cancer specimens can help predict prognosis. New drugs are being evaluated that may be useful in stopping breast cancer growth by preventing nourishment of the cancers by new blood vessels.

Benign breast tumors such as fibroadenomas or papillomas do not spread outside of the breast and are not life-threatening. Other tumors are malignant, which is another word for cancerous, and may become life-threatening.

Understanding some of the key words used to describe various types of breast cancer is important. An alphabetical list of terms, which includes the most important types of breast cancer, is provided below:

Adenocarcinoma: This is a general type of carcinoma that starts in glandular tissues anywhere in the body. There are several subtypes of adenocarcinoma which account for nearly all breast cancers.

Comedocarcinoma: In this type of ductal carcinoma in situ (DCIS), some of the cancer cells within ducts spontaneously begin to degenerate. This type of DCIS is more likely to recur locally after lumpectomy and may have a higher risk for being associated with invasive ductal carcinoma than other forms of DCIS.

Ductal carcinoma in situ (DCIS): Ductal carcinoma in situ is noninvasive breast cancer. Cancer cells fill the ducts but do not spread through the walls of the ducts into the fatty tissue of the breast. Nearly 100% of women diagnosed at this early stage of breast cancer may be cured. Only in the rarest circumstances can DCIS be detected by breast self-examination or clinical breast examination. The changes caused by DCIS usually can be seen by means of a screening mammography. With more women getting mammograms each year, the diagnosis of DCIS is becoming more common.

Infiltrating (or invasive) ductal carcinoma (IDC): Starting in a milk passage, or duct, of the breast, this cancer breaks through the wall of the duct and invades the fatty tissue of the breast. At this point, it has the potential to metastasize, or spread, to other parts of the body through the bloodstream and lymphatic system. Infiltrating ductal carcinoma is the most common type of breast cancer, accounting for about 80% of breast malignancies.

Infiltrating (or invasive) lobular carcinoma (ILC): ILC has arisen in the milk-producing glands and is invasive in the breast's fatty tissue. This cancer has the potential to spread (metastasize) elsewhere in the body. About 10% to 15% of invasive breast cancers are invasive lobular carcinomas. ILC is often difficult to detect by physical examination or even by mammography.

Inflammatory breast cancer: This rare type of invasive breast cancer accounts for about 1% of all breast cancers. It is an aggressive cancer that usually spreads rapidly to other parts of the body. Characteristically, it makes the skin over the breast look red and feel warm, causes it to thicken to the texture of an orange peel. Sometimes the breast develops ridges and small bumps that look like hives. These symptoms are caused by cancer cells blocking lymph vessels or channels in the skin over the breast.

In situ: This term is used to indicate an early stage of cancer in which a tumor is confined to the immediate area where it began. Specifically in breast cancer, in situ means that the cancer remains confined to ducts or lobules, and it has neither invaded surrounding fatty tissues in the breast nor spread to other organs in the body.

Lobular carcinoma in situ (LCIS): While not a cancer, LCIS, sometimes called lobular neoplasia, is sometimes classified as a type of non-invasive breast cancer. It begins in the milk-producing glands, but does not penetrate through the wall of the lobules. Women with LCIS are at increased risk of developing an invasive breast cancer over the long term in either breast. For this reason, it's important for women with LCIS to have a physical exam three times a year and an annual mammogram.

Medullary carcinoma: This special type of infiltrating breast cancer has a relatively well-defined, obvious boundary between tumor tissue and normal tissue. It accounts for about 5% of breast cancers. The outlook, or prognosis, for this kind of breast cancer is considered to be better than that of other types of infiltrating breast cancer.

Metastases: These are satellite tumors that indicate a breast cancer has spread from the site where it began (referred to as the **primary cancer**) to a lymph node or a distant organ, such as the lung or brain. In **micrometastasis**, (not to be confused with microcalcifications as noted below), the metastases are so small that they can be seen only under a microscope.

Microcalcifications: These are calcium deposits, often found in clusters by a mammogram. These deposits, sometimes called **calcifications**, are **neither cancer nor tumors**. But they are signs of changes within the breast, often merely due to aging, and they are very common. Because certain patterns of calcifications can be associated with cancer or benign breast disease, your medical team will want to monitor these changes. Follow-up may be either by periodic mammography or by biopsy, a procedure in which a sample of the breast tissue containing the calcium deposit is taken to test for cancer cells.

Mucinous carcinoma: This special type of infiltrating breast cancer is formed by mucus-producing cancer cells. The prognosis for mucinous carcinoma is considered to be better than for usual types of infiltrating breast cancer.

Node-positive (or negative) breast cancer: **Node-positive** means that the cancer has spread (metastasized) to the lymph nodes under the arm on the same side, which are called axillary nodes. **Node-negative** means that the biopsied lymph nodes are free of cancer. This is an indication that the cancer is less likely to recur.

Paget's disease of the nipple: This type of breast cancer starts in the milk passages, or ducts, and involves the skin of the nipple and can spread to the areola, the dark circle around the nipple. It is a rare type of breast cancer, occurring in only 1% of all cases. With Paget's disease of the nipple, there is usually a long history of crusting, scaly, red, inflamed tissue on the nipple and itching, oozing, burning, or bleeding. Using the fingertips, a lump may be detected within the breast. If no lump can be felt, the cancer generally has a good outcome, or prognosis. Paget's disease may be associated with in situ carcinoma or with infiltrating breast carcinoma (see above).

Phyllodes tumor: This very rare type of breast tumor forms from the connective tissue of the breast, in contrast to carci-

nomas which arise in the ducts or lobules. Phyllodes tumors are usually benign but rarely may be malignant. Benign phyllodes tumors are treated by removal, while malignant ones may metastasize (spread) and become life-threatening.
Scirrhous cancer: This is a breast carcinoma with a very hard texture. Some infiltrating ductal carcinomas and some infiltrating lobular carcinomas may have a scirrhous texture.
Tubular carcinomas: Accounting for about 2% of all breast cancers, tubular carcinomas are a special type of infiltrating breast carcinoma with a better outlook than the usual infiltrating ductal or lobular carcinomas.

References

1. M. Holcomb, and S. Safe, Inhibition of 7, 12-dimethylbenzanthracene-induced rat mammary tumor growth by 2,3,7,8-tetrachlorodibenzo-p-dioxin, *Cancer Letters* 82, 43-47, 1994.
2. W. Ganong, *Review of Medical Physiology*, p. 415, 1995, 17th edition, Appleton & Lange.
3. Y. Hirshaut and P.I. Pressman, *Breast Cancer, The Complete Guide*, 1992, Bantam Book.
4. L. Stryer, *Biochemistry*, p. 615, 1988, 3rd edition, W.H. Freeman and Company.
5. M. Holcomb, *International Toxicology*, p. 65, 1995, Western Printers.
6. *The Merck Manual*, Breast Cancer, 173, Breast Disorders, Section 14, Gynecology and Obstetrics, 16th edition, 1992, Merck.
7. National Institutes of Health, National Cancer Institute, *Chemotherapy and You, A Guide to Self-Help During Treatment*, NIH Publication, No. 95-1136, Revised July 1993, reprinted April 1995.
8. K.B. Horwitz and W.L. McGuire, Antiestrogens: Mechanisms of Action and Effects in Breast Cancer, in W.L. Guired, *Breast Cancer: Advances in Research and Treatment*, pp. 155-204, New York, 1978, Plenum Publishing Corp.
9. W. Ganong, *Review of Medical Physiology*, p. 417, 1995, 17th edition, Appleton & Lange.
10. R.R. Love, D.A. Wiebe, J.M. Feyzi, P.A. Newcomb and R.J. Chappell, Effects of Tamoxifen on Cardiovascular Risk Factors in Postmenopausal Women after 5 Years of Treatment, *Cancer Research Weekly*, p. 25(2), Nov. 21, 1994.
11. National Alliance of Breast Cancer Organization, April 1997, http://www.nabco.org/facts/genetics.html, New York, NY.
12. M. Segal and J.L. Willis, Progress Against Breast Cancer, An FDA Consumer Special Report, *Your Guide to Women's Health*, pp. 4-15,

September 1997, DHHS Publication No. (FDA) 97-1181, Department of Health & Human Services Public Health Service, Food and Drug Administration.

CHAPTER 3
Worldwide Learning

Women—and to a significantly lesser extent men—get breast cancer worldwide. The important thing we have learned about preventing death from breast cancer is the importance of early detection of the disease. Once the disease has traveled to other sites in the body, the treatments are usually more extensive and the undesirable side-effects from radiation, chemotherapy, hormone therapy or other treatments are temporarily unpleasant. Also, the health team selected can mean the difference between life, poor quality life, and death.

We have reviewed the scientific literature of studies or trials conducted in Germany, Italy, Japan, Canada, France, United Kingdom, India, Spain, the former Soviet Union, and the United States. The treatments for breast cancer in these countries are similar, but the quality of care and survival rates are different. Equally interesting is the varied treatment individual patients receive within a country. It is my impression from the literature that women in the upper-income group with an awareness of breast cancer self-examination and clinical exam have a higher probability of living once breast cancer is detected than lower-income women. Let's examine each country and get a better idea of the types of treatments available.

EUROPE

There is enormous variation in breast cancer treatment

practices throughout Europe. The Europe Against Cancer program has established a network of reference centers called the European Network of Reference Centres to establish quality assurance in mammography breast cancer screening. This is a great idea because in theory it insures that all women get a high quality mammography and the potential to detect breast cancer while it is still curable. In Europe mammography screening for breast cancer is recommended for women in the age group of 50 years and older. A two-view technique using a mediolateral oblique combined with a cranio-caudal projection is recommended for the initial screening examination. The incidence of breast cancer is relatively low in Southern and Eastern Europe when compared to the North and West. Approximately 75% of women in Europe with breast cancer are aged 50 or over. The increase in breast cancer death by 50% is because of the growth in the size of the effected population.[13]

GERMANY

Germany is a member of the European Union and has an excellent, well-structured health system. A complete and extensive booklet on the ways to detect cancer through the use of mammography techniques has been published by the European Commission. One translated abstract of a German article explained some of the history and treatments used for breast cancer. Again, we must state how important it is to detect breast cancer early.

For Germany, the treatment for breast cancer that has traveled to the liver can include surgery and chemotherapy treatments. The prognosis of survival rate of these women was rather unfavorable. The data indicates that from 1982-1991 42 patients were involved in a study to determine an appropriate treatment route. Post-operatively patients (27) received regional combined chemotherapy. The drugs used were 5-fluorouracil (1000 mg/12h/d/2d), Adriamycin (20 mg/12h/d/3d), and Mitomycin C (10 mg/2h/d/1d). An increase in survival rate was not seen in patients with partial liver resection with regional therapy or in patients with intraarterial chemotherapy. However, in exceptional cases a successful regional chemotherapy may be of significant benefit.[14]

ITALY

Italy is a member of the European Union. The only study we could locate deals with the movement of breast cancer from the breast to the bone.

In Italy doctors used disodium pamidronate (45 mg. infused over 1 hr. and repeated every 21 days) in breast cancer patients with bone metastases. This chemical did not induce sclerosis of lytic lesions from pretreated breast cancer.[15]

JAPAN

In Japan deaths from breast cancer are relatively low compared to Western countries. However, patterns of other types of cancer among Japanese is approaching that in Western countries.[16]

Pre-treatment (neoadjuvant chemotherapy) and after-surgery treatment (adjuvant chemotherapy) is used to control breast cancer. There is an increased life expectancy for breast cancer patients who get chemotherapy in increased dose intensity regimen. The dose of the chemotherapy agent and when it is given can determine the effectiveness of the treatment.[17]

If a breast tumor is small enough, it is removed and the breast is not significantly disfigured. The Japanese call the removal of a lump breast conserving treatment or BCT. For women to have BCT, the operation must (1) give the same control of breast cancer as a radical mastectomy, and (2) provide a clear cosmetic and psychological advantage to the patient. The general trend is to remove a good margin of healthy tissue with the lump. If the cancer is large, a large amount of breast may be removed (quadrantectomy) and a small dose of radiation used to provide adequate local control. While this may not meet the cosmetic and psychological goals, it may prevent the cancer from coming back. The overall treatments in Japan for breast cancer are surgical, radiological and chemotherapeutic techniques.[18]

Breast cancer that metastizes to bone may influence survival rate. Premenopausal or late postmenopausal status and longer disease-free intervals or no disease-free intervals may increase survival rate.[19]

CANADA

Treatment of breast cancer with systemic therapy significantly improves survival rates.

In 1974 no adjuvant systemic therapy was recommended.

In 1980 adjuvant chemotherapy was recommended for premenopausal women with node-positive disease.

In 1984 adjuvant chemotherapy was recommended for premenopausal women with lymph node or lymphatic, vacular or neural invasion unless tumors were negative for estrogen receptors.[20-21]

Patients requiring radiation treatment for breast cancer that involved lumpectomy have to wait 10 days in the Unites States and 43 days in Canada.

Patients having a lumpectomy requiring radiation treatment have to wait 10 days in the United States and 43 days in Canada. In general, cancer patients get faster radiotherapy in the United States than in Canada.

"The majority of radiation oncologists in both Canada and the USA regarded the delays reported by Canadian departments as medically unacceptable."[22]

FRANCE

In 1980 breast cancer represented 18% of all cancers in women worldwide. The worldwide incidence of breast cancer is increasing by 1.5% per annum. Breast cancer is influenced by geographical factors and by age.

In France, 19% of the cancer deaths are breast cancer and it is the commonest cause of cancer death in women.

Important indicators of potential for breast cancer:
　1) Age at menarche
　2) Age at menopause
　3) Parity
　4) Age at first pregnancy

The use of oral contraceptives and hormone replacement therapy for menopause *do not appear* to affect the development of malignant breast disease, except perhaps in certain sub-groups of patients (has not been confirmed).

Increased risk of breast cancer if there is a lot of fatty diet and excessive alcohol consumption and a family history of breast cancer.[23]

It is possible to inherit breast cancer from a family member. The highest risk was observed when a sister was affected by breast cancer. More genetic epidemiological studies are needed to define the mode of inheritance of the disease.[24]

In France radiotherapy is used to delay surgery or replace surgery when the breast cancer is inoperable. Radiotherapy is used for the local control of cancer.[25]

Thirty-two breast cancer patients had laparotomy to treat liver metastases from breast cancer. Patients treated with hepatectomy had a median survival at least three-fold that of patients treated with standard non-surgical treatment. There were confounding factors such as the lack of effective chemotherapy agents.[26]

UNITED KINGDOM

In the United Kingdom pre-treatment with chemo-endocrine agents was not recommended pre-surgery. There is a high rate of response to pre-treatment and a suggestion that there is a decrease in the requirement for mastectomy. However, the authors were waiting for the survival data from the National Surgical Adjuvant Breast and Bowel Project before making a recommendation.[27]

The importance of individual breast cancer treatments should be given more consideration. Pretreatment of breast cancer with the appropriate chemotherapy agents prior to surgery may increase the survival rate of individuals.[28]

History

In the United Kingdom the benefits of systemic treatment of breast cancer have been recognized for over a century.[29]

In the U.K. the different methods of treating breast cancer

affect the survival rate of individual patients by 12-23% at five years.

Interesting Facts
- Tumor assay for estrogen receptors are important
- Node invasion or not can determine treatment protocol
- Tumor size determines amount of breast removed
- C-erb B-2 and or p53 expression are chemo resistant *in vitro*
- Taxanes preferentially kill p53 deficient tumor cells[28]

Tamoxifen (20 mg/day) can cause potentially malignant changes in the endometrium of postmenopausal women. Transvaginal ultrasonography can be used to identify women who should have endometrial samples removed for microscopic analysis.

Out of 111 postmenopausal women (aged 46-71 years), 39% of women taking tamoxifen had histological evidence of an abnormal endometrium compared with 10% in the control group.[30]

INDIA

In India women usually go to the doctor when breast cancer is in its advanced stages. They do not live very long after the cancer is found. A few studies we were able to find confirmed these data.

Breast cancer is 20% of all female cancers in India. One study contained 100 patients with breast cancer. Most patients came to the hospital with advanced breast cancer. Some patients were excluded from this study. Only 20 patients were aware of breast cancer before onset of cancer.

Some 57 patients were from urban areas, 43 from rural areas. They were educated and had a family history of breast cancer.

Fine needle aspiration cytology was used in 50 patients and was diagnostic in 39.

17 out of 43 patients had inadequate operations. 27 out of 43 patients had faulty adjuvant therapy. The use of staging investigations was incomplete.[31]

Bone marrow biopsy, including bone marrow aspiration, immuno peroxidase staining or epithelial membrane antigen are good devices to help diagnosis of breast cancer metastasis to the bone in India.[32]

SPAIN

We reviewed one abstract from Spain that indicates the importance of early breast cancer detection.

31 breast cancer patients (Jan. 1988-Dec. 1990), average age 51. 9 years were examined and staged to determine the progress of the cancer.

Stage of Cancer	Percentage of Women in Group	*Survival Rate
1	41.9%	83.3%
2	29%	66%
3A	16.1%	40%
3B	12.8%	0%

*Total survival 48 months after diagnosis

Treatment was with modified radical mastectomy, radiation, and hormonal therapies. Systemic cytotoxic therapy was given to 77% of the patients.[33]

FORMER SOVIET UNION (FSU)

The awareness of the importance of early detection is known in Russia (FSU). However, we could not locate any survival data or indication that this principle is being applied. However, one study indicated that there is a correlation between effectiveness of therapy and size and number of metastatic nodes.[34]

UNITED STATES OF AMERICA

Our office is located in the United States of America. So we have available a significant amount of breast cancer information. Some of the scientific articles we reviewed are included in this summary. Also, we have included a discussion of mammography facilities available to the public in the United States.

Mammography Facilities

Congress enacted the Mammography Quality Standards Act of 1992. This act establishes requirements for the accreditation, certification and inspection of these facilities by the Food and Drug Administration (FDA).

All mammography facilities must be certified by FDA. The importance of technically qualified individuals to detect breast cancer early by the use of mammography can mean the difference between life and death. What we have learned from our worldwide review of breast cancer treatments is that the quality of mammography facilities varies widely, and women should be cautious on whom they select to perform these examinations.

Breast cancer is the most common cancer and the second leading cause of cancer death among women in the United States. (Lung cancer is the number one cancer killer.)

Breast Cancer* (Type)	5-Years Relative Survival Rates
Infiltrating duct carcinoma	79%
Lobular carcinoma	84%
Medullary carcinoma	82%
Mucinous (colloid) adenocarinoma	95%
Comedo carcinoma	87%
Paget's disease (nipple and other breast)	79%
Papillary carcinoma	95%
Tubular adenocarcinoma	96%
Inflammatory carcinoma	18%
Carcinomas in situ (all forms)	100%[35]

*Data from the Surveillance, Epidemiology and End Results program registry of the National Cancer Institute. 158,621 invasive and 10,639 in situ. 5-year relative survival rates.

Breast cancer is rare in men. About 1,000 men each year in the United States get breast cancer. Tumors from men are likely to be estrogen positive. Tumors are surgically removed and hormone, radiation, and cytotoxic therapies are used for treatment of the breast cancer.[36]

The survival rate, symptoms, clinical staging, and proposed treatments are the same for males as for women with breast cancer. (While this is not data from the United States, we have no reason to believe there is any significant difference in these data worldwide.)[37]

For women between the ages of 15 and 54 years, breast cancer is the most common cause of cancer-related death.

In Asian countries, where the incidence and mortality rates for breast cancer have been historically low, both have been increasing at a greater pace than in the industrialized West.

Breast cancer is usually diagnosed in later stages in developing countries. The mortality rates are much higher than in the U.S. or Western Europe.

Ovarian ablation prolonged disease-free and sometimes overall survival for premenopausal women with estrogen positive tumors.

The use of chemotherapy, hormone therapy or combination therapy or radiation should be evaluated on individual basis.

Women less than 50 years old, positive estrogen receptor, use tamoxifen, and women greater than 50 years old, postmenopausal with negative estrogen receptor do not usually get tamoxifen.[38]

Chemotherapy Drugs
Cyclophosphamine
Melphalan
Thiotepa
Methotreixate
5-fluorouracil
Prednisone
Melphalan
*Anthracycline-based
Doxorubicin
Epirubicin
Vincristine[38]   *Cardiac toxicity

Treatment with tamoxifen or CMF will affect the quality of life of a breast cancer patient, but this effect usually ends after treatment is completed.[39]

Older women (65-80) are not treated as often as younger women with radiation therapy.[40]

The use of high dose chemotherapy with bone marrow transplantation may provide a higher survival rate for women with breast cancer.[41]

Women treated with tamoxifen for five years post-surgery and one year of chemotherapy lived as long as those who were not treated with tamoxifen.

Tamoxifen does not appear to increase the lifespan of women treated for five years after initial treatment with surgery and one year of chemotherapy. However, estrogen node positive breast cancer women benefited from the treatment with tamoxifen post-surgery and one year of chemotherapy, but it was not statistically significant.[42]

The common terms used in the treatment of breast cancer with radiotherapy are descriptive of the repair system of some cells. -p53 protein = DNA damage repair. p53 and Bcl-2 = control of programmed cell death. Glutathione s-transferase [P1] [GST[ii]] enzyme = cellular detoxification.

Radiation therapy helps prevent local breast cancer relapse in node-negative patients with tumors that express elevated levels of the p53 or GST-[Pi] proteins, and little or no Bcl-2 protein. This is indirect evidence from two cohorts' studies.[43]

Women treated with chemotherapy drugs usually gain weight because of a decrease in physical activity and a slowing down in metabolism.

Chemotherapy agents used include:
    cyclophosphamide + doxorubicin + 5-fluorouracil
    cyclophosphamide + methotrexate + 5-fluorouracil
    [+ or -] doxorubicin
    cyclophosphamide + deoxorucin [+ or -] leucovorin
    methotrexate + 5-fluorouracil + leucovorin[44]

Data from Scotland and Sweden suggests that tamoxifen therapy can reduce the risk of heart attack (coronary heart disease). Results of this study indicated the death rate of tamoxifen treated patients from heart attacks was lower than non-treated patients, but not statistically significant.[45]

Breast cancer is not passed through breast milk. Women with breast cancer can usually breast-feed from the unaffected breast.

Breast feeding a child reduces a woman's chance of developing breast cancer later.

Silicone breast implants usually do not interfere with a woman's ability to nurse. Precautions should be taken to prevent implant leaks (potential esophagus damage to child).[46]

Disease-free state can be prolonged by the use of chemotherapy and hormonal therapy. For example, premenopausal nodal-positive patients can receive six cycles of CMF. Tamoxifen reduced overall tumor recurrence and mortality in postmenopausal estrogen receptor positive patients, but not significantly in estrogen negative patients.[47]

180,000 women get breast cancer each year in the United States. Systemic and local treatment is currently used to treat breast cancer.[48]

Hypothesis: For breast cancer to metastasize to the bone, it must proliferate, invade, migrate, survive and arrest in bone. This requires interaction with osteoclasts (theoretical).[49]

The most important risk factor for breast cancer is advancing age.

80% of women with breast cancer have none of the currently identified risk factors.

Breast conservation therapy (BCT), although highly recommended for "lump" removal, is not used in all locations in the USA.

The author suggests that education of both the doctor and the patient about BCT be done to make them aware of the current management of breast cancer.[50]

There is a four to five-fold variation in breast cancer incidence rates across different countries.

The lowest rate of breast cancer is in Asia, and the highest rates are observed in western Europe and North America. 50-60% increase in reported breast cancer in Japan, Singapore and Hungary.[51]

The relationship between breast cancer and nutrition needs to be investigated.[52]

The presence of breast cancer can go undetected if the mammogram and cytology tests suggest cancer cells are not present.[53]

The data indicates that neither BRCA1 or p53 is a major susceptible gene in Japanese familial breast cancer. In two site-specific breast cancer families, the BRCA1 gene was detected.[54]

Lobular carcinoma in situ (LCIS) and ductal carcinoma in situ (DCIS) are non-invasive breast cancers. The increased ability to detect these cancers with mammography has caused more cases of non-invasive breast cancer (to be discussed).[55]

Other non-related studies show the importance of genetics. This group of scientists identified three regions of amplification and nine chromosomal arms with deletions in the genorme.

Recent works show a commonly deleted region between D 17 S846 and D 17 S746 that is approximately 0.5-1.0 Mb centromeric to the newly described BRCA1 gene.[56]

Pregnancy

Pregnancy does not stimulate the growth of breast cancer. No therapeutic justification exists for abortion.

Treatment should be altered or delayed because of pregnancy.

After breast cancer treatment, a two-year waiting period prior to becoming pregnant is appropriate. The management of breast cancer in pregnancy should be handled by many experts including the breast surgeon, obstetrician, breast counselor, medical oncologist and radiotherapist.[57]

Biology of Cancer

Normal breast epithelium must undergo a series of complex, multi-step processes to become cancerous. At some point in the process there could be a decrease in the tumor suppressor gene activity, an increase of oncogene activity, or loss of ability to respond to hormonal growth regulatory signals.[58]

Chemotherapy

For some 35 years chemotherapy has been a major management technique used to control breast cancer. Chemotherapy is given before surgery and increases survival rate 50% to 70%. As an adjuvant treatment for both node positive and node negative breast cancer, chemotherapy improves overall and relapse-free survival rate regardless of reproductive state (pre or post-menopause).

Chemotherapy agents used include alkylizing agents, 5-fluoro-uracil, anthracyclines and methotrexate used in combinations.

As of 1994, new cytostatic agents in Phase I and Phase II trials include vinorelbine and taxoid agents.

The use of medullan growth factors autografting with bone marrow and circulating stem cells have made it possible to increase the amount of chemotherapy agents used in the treatment of breast cancer.[59]

Animal Data

A comparison of the beagle dog breast cancer model with the lifetime breast cancer rate of Japanese and U.S. white men and women suggest there is a linkage between the adult cancer mortality regardless of different patterns of cancer types and environments.[60]

Human Data

Tamoxifen (20 mg) or toremifene (60 mg) produces comparable estrogenic effects in the uterus and vagina of breast cancer patients (N = 31). Polyps and fibroids may increase in size or develop.[61]

Breast cancer, adenocarcinoma, rarely travel to the uterus. However, if it does spread to the uterus or cervix, the patient has a high probability of death.[62]

Stage I or II invasive breast cancer cannot be adequately treated with only conservative surgery. The use of conservative surgery and radiotherapy will provide more protection from cancer recurrence.

The use of conservative surgery alone in clinical studies is "reasonable" if the patient is adequately informed of the risks.[63]

The use of iridium-192 high-dose rate implantation can kill potentially harmful cells and increase the amount of radiation to the site by 10 Gy if used with external-beam irradiation. (This data is from Austria, but may be of interest to USA professionals.)[64]

Patients undergoing radiation treatment may suffer emotional distress. Therapy in the form of cognitive behavioral treatment and social support may be helpful when compared with no treatment.[65]

The synthetic tetracycline, doxycycline, inhibits migration of human MDA-MB-435 breast adenocarcinoma cells through a reconstituted basement membrane. Doxycycline diminishes the growth of this breast cancer cell line and decreases its gelatinolytic activity.[66]

Breast cancer that spreads to other parts of the body accounts for 18% of cancer deaths among women in the U.S.

Autologous bone marrow transplantation should be considered for a select number of patients with metastatic breast cancer. Relapses of breast cancer can occur after treatment.[67]

A recommendation of *not* conducting routine bone scans for follow-up of patients with Stage I-II breast cancer unless symptoms suggest bone metastases.[68]

Once an insurance company determines that a clinical trial involving chemotherapy and autologous bone marrow transplantation for breast cancer is not necessary, a significant barrier to obtaining treatment occurs.

In some cases a patient may have to hire an attorney to gain coverage.[69]

Limited selected data indicate certain subgroups of breast cancer patients with metastatic liver disease may benefit from aggressive regional therapy with chemotherapy agents like 5-FU, adriamycin, methotrexate and cytoxan.[70]

References
13. European Guidelines for Quality Assurance in Mammography Screening, 2nd ed., Europe Against Cancer, European Commission, June 1996, Editors Dr. C.J.M. de Wolf and Dr. N.M. Perry, Luxembourg: Office for Official Publication of the European Communities.
14. Lorenz, M., Wiesner, J., Staib-Sebler, E., Encke, A., Regional Therapy Breast Cancer Liver Metastases, *Zentralbl Chir* 120: 10, 7886-90, 1995.
15. M. Colleuni, Bochicchio, A.M., Nole, F., Bajetta, E., Disodium pamidronate in the treatment of bone metastases from breast cancer, *Tumor*: 79:5, 340-2, Oct. 31, 1993.
16. S. Tominaga, Recent Trends in Cancer in Japan and the World, Gan To Kagaku Ryoho 22:1, 1-8, Jan. 1995.
17. M. Fukuoka, Tsuchiya, R., Principles for adjuvant and neoadjuvant chemotherapy, Gun To Kagaku Ryoho, 21, Suppl 3: 333-7, Oct. 1994.
18. M. Noguchi, Miyazaki, I., Breast conserving surgery and radiation in the treatment of operable breast cancer, *Int. Surg.*, 79:2, 142-7, Apr.-Jun. 1994.
19. K. Yamashita, H. Koyama and H. Inaji, Prognostic significance of bone metastasis from breast cancer, *Clin. Orthop.* 312, 89-94, March 1995.
20. I. A. Olivotto, Adjuvant systemic therapy and survival after breast cancer, New England Journal of Medicine 1994; 330:805-810.
21. JAMA, The Journal of the American Medical Association, V. 273, N. 17, p. 1318R(1), May 3, 1995.
22. W.J. Mackillop, Zhou, Y., Quirt, C.F., A comparison of delays in the treatment of cancer with radiation in Canada and the United States, *Int. J. Radiat. Oncol. Biol. Phys.* 32:2, 531-9, May 15, 1995.
23. J. M. Ferrero, Namer, M., Epidemiology of cancer of the breast (Epidemiologie du cancer du sein), *Arch Anat Cytol. Pathol.* 42:5, 198-205, 1994.

24. N. Andrieu, Clavel F., Gairard B., Piana L., Bremond A., Lansac J., Flamant, R., Renaud, R., Familial risk of breast cancer in a French case-control study, *Cancer Detect Prev.* 18:3, 163-9, 1994.
25. F. Baillet, Radiotherapy—an alternative to surgery in the treatment of breast cancer, *Chirurgie* 120: 6-7, 343-7; discussion 347-8, -95, 1994.
26. D. Elias, P.H. Lassen, D. Montrucolli, S. Bonvallot, and M. Spielman, Hepatectomy for liver metastases from breast cancer, *Eur. J. Surg. Oncol.* 21:5, 510-3, Oct. 1995.
27. T.J. Powles, Hickish, T.F., Makris, A., Ashley, S.E., O'Brien, M.E., Tidy, V.A., Casey, S., Nash, A.G., Sacks, N., Cosgrove, D. et al, Randomized trial of chemoendocrine therapy started before or after surgery for treatment of primary breast cancer, *J. Clin. Oncol.* 13:3, 547-52, March 1995.
28. R. Epstein, Treating breast cancer before surgery: cure rates could be improved by better matching of drugs to disease. British Medical Journal, Nov. 30, 1996, v. 313, n. 7069, p. 1345(2).
29. G.T. Beatson, On the treatment of inoperable cases of carcinoma of the mamma: Suggestions for a new method of treatment, with illustrative cases. Cancer, 1996; II: 104-7, 162-5.
30. R. P. Kedar, Bourne, T.H., Powles, T.J., Collins, W.P., Ashley, S.E., Cosgrove, P.O., Campbell, S. Effects of tamoxifen on uterus and ovaries of postmenopausal women in a randomized breast cancer prevention trial, Lancet 343:8909, 1318-21, May 1994.
31. A.K. Goel, V. Seen, N.K. Shukla, and V. Raina, Breast cancer presentation at a regional cancer centre, *Natl. Med. J. India*, 8:1, 6-9, Jan.-Feb. 1995.
32. D. Basu, T. Singh, R.N. Shinghal, Micrometastasis in bone marrow in breast cancer. Indian J. Pathol. Microbiol. 37:2, 159-64, April 1994.
33. J. L. Caballero, B. Rios, Breast cancer (cancer de mama), *Rev. Med. Panama* 20:1-2, 50-3, Jan.-May 1995.
34. E. K. Voznyi, Meshcheriakova, N.G., Buianov, S.S., Dobrovolskaia, N.I., Diagnosis and therapy of liver metastasis of breast cancer, *Vopr. Onkol.* 40: 7-12, 353-6, 1994.
35. J. W. Berg, R. V. Hutter, Breast Cancer 75:1 Suppl, 257-69, Jan. 1, 1995.
36. J. R. Hecht, Winchester, D.J., Male breast cancer, Am. J. Clin. Pathol., 102:4, Suppl 1, 525-30, Oct. 1994.
37. I. Veys, Nogaret, J.M., Male breast cancer (Le cancer du sein au masculin), *Rev. Med. Brux*, 16:6, 394-6, Dec. 1995.
38. G. N. Hortobagyi and A.U. Buzdar, Current status of adjuvant systemic therapy for primary breast cancer: progress and controversy,

July-August 1995, v. 45, n. 4, p. 199 (28).
39. C. Hurny, J. Bernhard, A.J. Coates, M. C-Gertsch, H.F. Peterson, R.D. Gelber, J.F. Forbes, C-M. Rudenstam, E. Simanchi, D. Crivellari, A. Goldhirsch, and H-J. Senn. The Lancet, May 11, 1996, v. 347, n. 9011, p. 1279(6).
40. Adjuvant radiation in older cancer patients depends on age, other diseases. *Cancer Weekly Plus*, June 17, 1996, p. 9(1).
41. S.L. Goldberg, T.R. Klumpp and K.F. Mangan, Why consider bone marrow transplantation in breast cancer? *American Family Physician*, Sept. 1, 1996, v. 54, n. 3, p. 856(3).
42. D.C. Tormey, R. Gray and H.C. Falkson, Postchemotherapy adjuvant tamoxifen therapy beyond five years in patients with lymph node-positive breast cancer, *Journal of the National Cancer Institute*, Dec. 18, 1996, v. 88, n. 24, p. 1828(6).
43. R. Silvestrhi, S. Veneroni, E. Benini, M.G. Daidone, A. Luisi, M. Leutner, A. Mauclone, R. Kenda, R. Zucali, and U. Veronesi. Expression of p53, gluthathione s-transferose -pi, and Bc1-2 proteins and benefit from adjuvant radiotherapy in breast cancer.
44. W.D. Wahnefried, V. Hare, M.R. Conaway, K. Havlin, B.K. Rimer, G. McElveen, and E.P. Winer, Reduced rates of metabolism and decreased physical activity in breast cancer patients receiving adjuvant chemotherapy, *American Journal of Clinical Nutrition*, May 1997, v. 65, n. 5, p. 1495(7).
45. J.P. Costantino, L.H. Kuller, D.G. Ives, B. Fisher and J. Digram, Coronary heart disease mortality and adjuvant tamoxifen therapy, *Journal of the National Cancer Institute*, June 4, 1997, v. 89, n. 11, p. 776(7).
46. *Your Guide to Women's Health*, Third Edition, HE 20, 4010/4 W84/2.
47. W. Jonat, H. Eidtmann, Chemotherapy and hormone therapy in breast carcinoma (Die chemo und die Hormontherapie des mammakarzinoms), *Schweiz Rundsch Med Prax* 84: 13, 386-9, Mar. 28, 1995.
48. B.A. Overmoyer, Chemotherapy in the management of breast cancer, *Cleve Clin. J. Med.* 62:1, 36-50, Jan.-Feb. 1995.
49. T. Yoneda, A. Sasaki, and G.R. Mundy, Osteolytic bone metastasis in breast cancer, *Breast Cancer Res. Treat* 32: 1, 73-84, 1994.
50. D.J. Marchant, Contemporary management of breast cancer, *Obstet. Gynecol. Clin. North Am.* 21:4, 555-60, Dec. 1994.
51. G. Ursin, L. Bernstein, M.C. Pike, Breast Cancer, *Cancer Surv.* 19-20: 241-64, 1994.
52. Nutrition and breast cancer, *Oncology*, Hunting, T., 71-5; discussion 76, 79-80, Dec. 1993.
53. N.C. Davis, J.J. Herron, A missed breast cancer, *Aust. N.Z. J. Surg.*

65:7, 536-7, July 1995.
54. T. Fukutomi, Inoue R., Ushijima, T., Toyoda, M., Familial breast cancer, Nippon Rinsho 53: 11, 2764-8, Nov. 1995.
55. M. Rebner, Roju U., Non-invasive breast cancer, *Radiology* 190:3, 623-31, Mar. 1994.
56. C.S. Cropp, Mutations in breast cancer, *Cancer Lett* 90: 1, 51-6, Mar. 23, 1995.
57. J.H. Isaacs, Cancer of the breast in pregnancy, *Surg. Clin. North Am.* 75: 1, 47-51, Feb. 1995.
58. K. Hoskins, Weber, B.L., The biology of breast cancer, *Curr Opin. Oncol.* 6:6, 554-9, Nov. 1994.
59. J.L. Breau, Chemotherapy in the management of breast cancer (La chimiotherapie dane ie traitement du cancer du sein), *Chirurgie* 120: 6-7, 354-6, 95, 1994.
60. R.E. Alberg, Benjamin S.A., Shubla, K., Life span and cancer mortality in the beagle dog and humans, *Mech Age. Dev.* 74: 3, 149-59, June 1994.
61. E. Tomas, Kauppila, A., Blanco, G., Apaja-Sarkkinen, M., Laatikainen, T., Comparison between the effects of tamoxifen and toremifene to the uterus in postmenopausal breast cancer patients, *Gynecol. Oncol.* 59:2, 261-6, Nov. 1995.
62. J.B. Taxy, Trujillo, Y.P., Breast cancer metastatic to the uterus, clinical manifestations of a rare event, *Arch. Pathol. Lab. Med.* 118:8, 819-21, Aug. 1994.
63. A. Recht, Houlihan, M.J., Conservation surgery without radiotherapy in the treatment of patients with early-stages invasive breast cancer, a review, *Ann Surg.* 222; 1, 9-18, July 1995.
64. J. Hammer, Seewald, D.H., Track C., Zoidl, J.P., Labeck, W., Breast cancer: primary treatment with external-beam radiation therapy and high-dose-rate iridium implantation, *Radiology* 193:2, 573-7, Nov. 1994.
65. R.L. Evans, Connis, R.T., Comparison of brief group therapies for depressed cancer patients receiving radiation treatments, *Public Health Rep.* 110:3, 306-11, May-June 1995.
66. R.S. Fife, Slenge, G.W., Jr., Effects of doxycycline on *in vitro* growth, migration, and gelatinase activity of breast carcinoma cells, *J. Lab. Clin. Med.* 125: 3, 407-11, March 1995.
67. R.A. Saez, Selby, G.B., Slease, R.B., Epstein, R.B., Mandanas, R.A., Confer, D.L., Autologous bone marrow transplantation for metastatic breast cancer, *J. Okla State Med. Association*, 87:9, 405-10, Sept. 1994.
68. K.A. Wikenheiser, Silberstein, E.G., Bone scintigraphy screening in stage I-II breast cancer: is it cost-effective? *Cleve. Clin. J. Med.* 63:1, 43-7, Jan.-Feb. 1996.

69. W.P. Peters, Rogers, M.C., Variation in approval by insurance companies of coverage for autologous bone marrow transplantation for breast cancer, *New England Journal Medicine* 330:7, 473-7, Feb. 17, 1994.
70. S. Schneebaum, Walker, M.J., Young, D., Farrar, W.B., Minton, J.P., The regional treatment of liver metastases from breast cancer, *J. Surg. Oncol.* 55: 1, 26-31; discussion 32, Jan. 1994.

Appendix

CHEMOTHERAPY AND YOU: A GUIDE TO SELF-HELP DURING TREATMENT

National Institutes of Health
National Cancer Institute

About This Booklet

This booklet will help you, your family, and your friends understand chemotherapy, the use of drugs to treat cancer. It will answer many of the questions you may have about this method of cancer treatment. It also will show you how you can help yourself during chemotherapy.

Taking care of yourself during chemotherapy is important for several reasons. For one thing, it can lessen some of the physical side effects you may have from your treatment. As you will see, some simple tips can make a big difference in how you feel. But the benefits of self-help aren't just physical; they're psychological, too. Knowing some ways to take care of yourself can give your emotions a boost at a time when you may be feeling that much of what's happening to you is out of your control. This feeling can be easier to deal with when you discover how you can contribute to your own well-being, in partnership with your doctors and nurses.

Chemotherapy and You will help you become an informed partner in your care. Remember, though, it is only a guide. Self-help is never a substitute for professional medical care. Be sure to ask your doctor and nurse any questions you may have about chemotherapy, and tell them about any side effects you may have.

You will find several helpful sections at the back of this booklet. The section on "Paying for Chemotherapy" gives you information about insurance and other payment methods. The section called "Resources" tells you how to get more information about cancer and how to find many services available to cancer patients and their families. The "Glossary" explains many terms related to cancer and chemotherapy. Words printed in **bold** are defined in the Glossary.

Finally, the page labeled "Notes" can be used to jot down ideas you want to remember or questions you want to ask your doctor or nurse.

This edition of *Chemotherapy and You* does not include the tear-out cards for drug information that were in previous versions. A free series of fact sheets on anticancer drugs is available from the National Cancer Institute. (See "Resources.")

[Note by author of International Breast Cancer Treatment: The free series of fact sheets on anticancer drugs was replaced. A person interested in getting information of a drug(s) should call 1-800-4CANCER.]

UNDERSTANDING CHEMOTHERAPY

What is Chemotherapy?

Chemotherapy is the use of drugs to treat cancer. The drugs often are called "anticancer" drugs.

How Does Chemotherapy Work?

Normal cells grow and die in a controlled way. But **cancer** occurs when cells become abnormal and keep dividing and forming more cells without control or order. Anticancer drugs destroy cancer cells by stopping them from growing or multiplying at one or more points in their life cycle. Because some drugs work better together than alone, chemotherapy often may consist of more than one drug. This is called **combination chemotherapy**.

In addition to chemotherapy, other methods sometimes are used to treat cancer. For example, your doctor may recommend that you have surgery to remove a tumor or to relieve certain symptoms that may be caused by your cancer. You also may receive **radiation therapy** to treat your cancer or its symptoms. Sometimes, as described below, your doctor may suggest a combination of chemotherapy, surgery, and/or radiation therapy. (See page 4.)

Other types of drugs may be used to treat your cancer. These may include certain drugs that can block the effect of hormones. Doctors also may use **biological therapy** to boost the body's natural defenses against cancer.

What Can Chemotherapy Achieve?
Depending on the type of cancer and its stage of development, chemotherapy can be used:
- To cure cancer.
- To keep the cancer from spreading.
- To slow the cancer's growth.
- To kill cancer cells that may have spread to other parts of the body from the original tumor.
- To relieve symptoms that may be caused by the cancer.

Chemotherapy also can help people live more comfortably; this is known as **palliative** care.

Will Chemotherapy Be My Only Treatment for Cancer?
Sometimes chemotherapy is the only therapy a patient receives. More often, however, chemotherapy is used in addition to surgery and/or radiation therapy; when it is used for this purpose it is called **adjuvant therapy**. There are several reasons why chemotherapy may be given in addition to other treatment methods. For instance, chemotherapy may be used to shrink a tumor before surgery or radiation therapy. It also may be used after surgery and/or radiation therapy to help destroy any cancer cells that may remain.

Which Drugs Will I Get?
Your doctor decides which drug or drugs will work best for you. The decision depends on what kind of cancer you have, where it is, the extent of its growth, how it is affecting your normal body functions, and your general health.

Your doctor also may suggest that you join a clinical trial for chemotherapy, or you may want to bring up this option with your doctor. Clinical trials are carefully designed research studies that test promising new cancer treatments. Patients who take part in research may be the first to benefit from improved treatment methods. These patients also can make an important contribution to medical care because the results of these studies may help many people. Patients participate in clinical trials only if they choose to and are free to withdraw at any time.

To learn more about clinical trials, call the National Cancer Institute's Cancer Information Service and ask for the booklet What Are Clinical Trials All About? You also may want to ask about the videotape "Patient to Patient: Cancer Clinical Trials and You." This videotape can put to rest fears you may have about taking part in clinical trials. The Cancer Information Service can be reached by dialing I -800-4-CANCER (1-800-422-6237).

Where Will I Get Chemotherapy?

You may get your chemotherapy at home, in your doctor's office, in a clinic, in your hospital's outpatient department, or in a hospital. The choice of where you get chemotherapy depends on which drug or drugs you are getting, your hospital's policies, and your doctor's preferences. When you first start chemotherapy, you may need to stay at the hospital for a short time so that your doctor can watch the medicine's effects closely and make any adjustments that are needed.

How Often Will I Get Chemotherapy, And How Long Will I Get It?

How often—and for how long—you get chemotherapy depends on the kind of cancer you have, the goals of the treatment, the drugs that are used, and how your body responds to them. You may get chemotherapy every day, every week, or every month. Chemotherapy is often given in on-and-off cycles that include rest periods so that your body has a chance to build healthy new cells and regain its strength. Your doctor should be able to estimate how long you will be getting chemotherapy.

Whatever schedule your doctor prescribes, it is very important to stay with it. Otherwise, the anticancer drugs might not have their desired effect. If you miss a treatment session or skip a dose of medication, contact your doctor for instructions about what to do.

Sometimes, your doctor may delay a treatment based on the results of certain blood tests. (See pages 18-22.) Your doctor will let you know what to do during this time and when it's okay to start your treatment sessions again.

How Will I Get Chemotherapy?

Depending on the type of cancer you have and the drug or drugs you are getting, your chemotherapy may be given in one or more of the following ways:

- Into a vein (**intravenously, or IV**). You will get the drug through a thin needle inserted into a vein, usually on your hand or lower arm. Another way to get IV chemotherapy is by means of a **catheter**, a thin tube that is placed into a large vein in your body and remains there as long as it is needed. This type of catheter is known as a **central venous catheter**. Sometimes, a central venous catheter is attached to a **port**, a small plastic or metal container placed surgically under the skin.
- By mouth (**orally, or PO**) in pill, capsule, or liquid form. You will swallow the drug, just as you do many other medications.
- Into a muscle (**intramuscularly, or IM**), under the skin (**subcutaneously, or SQ or SC**), or directly into a cancerous area in the skin (**intralesionally, or IL**). You will get an injection with a needle.
- Topically. The medication will be applied onto the skin.

Chemotherapy also may be delivered to specific areas of the body using a catheter (or a catheter plus a port). Catheters may be placed directly into the spinal fluid, abdominal cavity, bladder, or liver. Your doctor or nurse may use specific terms when talking about certain types of catheters. For example, an **intrathecal (IT)** catheter is used to deliver drugs into the spinal fluid. **Intracavitary (IC)** catheters can be placed in the abdomen, pelvis, or chest.

Two kinds of pumps—external and internal— may be used to control the rate of delivery of chemotherapy. External pumps remain outside of the body. Some are portable and allow a person to move around while the pump is in use. Other external pumps are not portable and may restrict activity. Internal pumps are placed surgically inside the body, usually right under the skin. They contain a small reservoir (storage area) that delivers the drugs into the catheter. Internal pumps allow people to go about most of their daily activities.

Does Chemotherapy Hurt?

Getting chemotherapy by mouth, on the skin, or by injection generally feels the same as taking other medications by these methods. Having an IV started usually feels like having blood drawn for a blood test. Some people feel a coolness or other unusual sensation in the area of the injection when the IV is started. Report these feelings to your doctor or nurse. Be sure that you also report any pain, burning, or discomfort that occurs during or after an IV treatment.

Many people have little or no trouble having the IV needle in their hand or lower arm. However, if a person has a hard time for any reason, or if it becomes difficult to insert the needle into a vein for each treatment, it may be possible to use a central venous catheter or port. This avoids repeated insertion of the needle into the vein.

Central venous catheters and ports cause no pain or discomfort if they are properly placed and cared for, although a person usually is aware that they are there. It is important to report any pain or discomfort with a catheter or port to your doctor or nurse.

Can I Take Other Medicines While I Am Getting Chemotherapy?

Some medicines may interfere with the effects of your chemotherapy. That is why you should take a list of all your medications to your doctor before you start chemotherapy. Your list should include the name of each drug, how often you take it, the reason you take it, and the dosage. Remember to include over-the-counter drugs such as laxatives, cold pills, pain relievers, and vitamins. Your doctor will tell you if you should stop taking any of these medications before you start chemotherapy. After your treatments begin, be sure to check with your doctor before taking any new medicines or stopping the ones you already are taking.

Will I Be Able to Work During Chemotherapy?

Most people are able to continue working while they are being treated with anticancer drugs. It may be possible to schedule your treatments late in the day or right before the weekend, so they interfere with work as little as possible.

If your chemotherapy makes you very tired, you might want to think about adjusting your work schedule for a while. Speak with your employer about your needs and wishes at this time. You may be able to agree on a part-time schedule, or perhaps you can do some of your work at home.

Under Federal and state laws, some employers may be required to allow you to work a flexible schedule to meet your treatment needs. To find out about your on-the-job protections, check with your local American Cancer Society, a social worker, or your congressional or state representative. The National Cancer Institute's publication *Facing Forward: A Guide for Cancer Survivors* also has information on work-related concerns.

How Will I Know If My Chemotherapy Is Working?

Your doctor and nurse will use several methods to measure how well your treatments are working. You will have frequent physical exams, blood tests, scans, and x-rays. Don't hesitate to ask the doctor about the test results and what they show about your progress.

While tests and exams can tell a lot about how chemotherapy is working, side effects tell very little. (Side effects—such as nausea or hair loss—occur because chemotherapy harms some normal cells as well as cancer cells.) Sometimes people think that if they don't have side effects, the drugs aren't working, or that, if they do have side effects, the drugs are working well. But side effects vary so much from person to person, and from drug to drug, that having them or not having them usually isn't a sign of whether the treatment is effective.

If you do have side effects, there is a lot you can do to help relieve them. The next section of this booklet describes some of the most common side effects of chemotherapy and gives you some hints for coping with them.

COPING WITH SIDE EFFECTS

If you have questions about side effects, you are not alone. Before chemotherapy starts, most people are concerned about whether they will have side effects and, if so, what they will be like. Once treatments begin, people who have side effects want to know the best ways to cope with them. This section will answer some of your questions.

If you are reading this section before you start chemotherapy, you may feel overwhelmed by the wide range of side effects it describes. But remember: Every person doesn't get every side effect, and some people get few, if any. In addition, the severity of side effects varies greatly from person to person. Whether you have a particular side effect, and how severe it will be, depends on the kind of chemotherapy you get and how your body reacts. Be sure to talk to your doctor and nurse about which side effects are most likely to occur with your chemotherapy, how long they might last, how serious they might be, and when you should seek medical attention for them.

What Causes Side Effects?

Because cancer cells grow and divide rapidly, anticancer drugs are made to kill fast-growing cells. But certain normal, healthy cells also multiply quickly, and chemotherapy can affect these cells, too. When it does, side effects may result. The fast-growing, normal cells most likely to be affected are blood cells forming in the bone marrow and cells in the digestive tract, reproductive system, and hair follicles. Anticancer drugs also can damage cells of the heart, kidney, bladder, lungs, and nervous system. The most common side effects of chemotherapy include nausea and vomiting, hair loss, and fatigue.

Other common side effects include an increased chance of bleeding, getting an infection, or developing anemia. (See pages 18 - 22.) These side effects result from changes in blood cells during chemotherapy.

How Long Do Side Effects Last?

Most normal cells recover quickly when chemotherapy is over, so most side effects gradually disappear after treatment ends, and the healthy cells have a chance to grow normally. The time it takes to get over some side effects and regain energy varies from person to person. How soon you will feel better depends on many factors, including your overall health and the kinds of drugs you have been taking.

While many side effects go away fairly rapidly, certain ones may take months or years to disappear completely. Sometimes the side effects can last a lifetime, as when chemotherapy causes permanent damage to the heart, lungs, kidneys, or reproductive organs. And certain types of chemotherapy occasionally may cause delayed effects, such as a second cancer, that show up many years later.

It is important to remember that many people have no long-term problems due to chemotherapy. It also is reassuring to know that doctors are making great progress in preventing some of chemotherapy's more serious side effects. For instance, they are using many new drugs and techniques that increase chemotherapy's powerful effects on cancer cells while decreasing its harmful effects on the body's healthy cells.

The side effects of chemotherapy can be unpleasant, but they must be measured against the treatment's ability to destroy cancer. People getting chemotherapy sometimes become discouraged about the length of time their treatment is taking or the side effects they are having. If that happens to you, talk to your doctor. It may be that your medication or the treatment schedule can be changed. Or your doctor may be able to suggest ways to reduce side effects or make them easier to tolerate. Remember though, your doctor will not ask you to continue treatments unless the expected benefits outweigh any problems you might have.

On the pages that follow, you will find suggestions for dealing with some of the more common side effects of chemotherapy.

Nausea and Vomiting

Chemotherapy can cause nausea and vomiting by affecting the stomach, the area of the brain that controls vomiting, or both. This reaction to chemotherapy varies from person to person and from drug to drug. For example, some people never vomit or feel nauseous. Others feel mildly nauseated most of the time, while some become severely nauseated for a limited time during or after a treatment. Their symptoms may start soon after a treatment or hours later. They may feel sick for just a few hours or for about a day. Be sure to tell your doctor or nurse if you are very nauseated and/or have vomited for more than a day or if your nausea is so bad that you cannot even keep liquids down.

Nausea and vomiting almost always can be controlled or at least lessened. If you experience this side effect, your doctor can choose from a range of drugs known as **antiemetics**, which help curb nausea and vomiting. Different drugs work for different people, and it may be necessary to use more than one drug to get relief. Don't give up. Continue to work with your doctor and nurse to find the drug or drugs that work best for you.

You can also try the following ideas:

- Avoid big meals so your stomach won't feel too full. Eat small meals throughout the day, instead of one, two, or three large meals.
- Drink liquids at least an hour before or after mealtime, instead of with your meals.
- Eat and drink slowly.
- Stay away from sweet, fried, or fatty foods.
- Eat foods cold or at room temperature so you won't be bothered by strong smells.
- Chew your food well for easier digestion.
- If nausea is a problem in the morning, try eating dry foods like cereal, toast, or crackers before getting up. (Don't try this if you have mouth or throat sores or if you are troubled by a lack of saliva.)
- Drink cool, clear, unsweetened fruit juices, such as apple or grape juice, or light-colored sodas, such as ginger ale, that have lost their fizz.
- Suck on ice cubes, mints, or tart candies. (Don't use tart candies if you have mouth or throat sores.)
- Try to avoid odors that bother you, such as cooking smells, smoke, or perfume.
- Prepare and freeze meals in advance for days when you don't feel like cooking.
- Rest in a chair after eating, but don't lie flat for at least 2 hours after you've finished your meal.
- Wear loose-fitting clothes.
- Breathe deeply and slowly when you feel nauseated.
- Distract yourself by chatting with friends or family members, listening to music, or watching a movie or TV show.

- Use relaxation techniques. (See pages 43-46.)
- Avoid eating for at least a few hours before treatment if nausea usually occurs during chemotherapy.

Hair Loss

Hair loss (**alopecia**) is a common side effect of chemotherapy, but it doesn't always happen. Your doctor can tell you whether hair loss is likely to occur with the drug or drugs you are taking. When hair loss does occur, the hair may become thinner or may fall out entirely. The hair usually grows back after the treatments are over. Some people even start to get their hair back while they are still having treatments. In some cases, hair may grow back in a different color or texture.

Hair loss can occur on all parts of the body, not just the head. Facial hair, arm and leg hair, underarm hair, and pubic hair all may be affected.

Hair loss usually doesn't happen right away; more often, it begins after a few treatments. At that point, hair may fall out gradually or in clumps. Any hair that is still growing may become dull and dry.

To care for your scalp and hair during chemotherapy:
- Use mild shampoos.
- Use soft hair brushes.
- Use low heat when drying your hair.
- Don't use brush rollers to set your hair.
- Don't dye your hair or get a permanent.
- Have your hair cut short. A shorter style will make your hair look thicker and fuller. It also will make hair loss easier to manage if it occurs.
- Use a sunscreen, sunblock, hat, or scarf to protect your scalp from the sun if you lose a lot of the hair on your head.

Some people who lose all or most of their hair choose to wear turbans, scarves, caps, wigs, or hairpieces. Others leave their head uncovered. Still others switch back and forth, depending on whether they are in public or at home with friends and family members. There are no "right" or "wrong" choices; do whatever feels comfortable for you.

Here are some tips if you choose to cover your head:
- Get your wig or hairpiece before you lose a lot of hair. That way, you can match your natural color and current hair

style if you wish. You may be able to buy a wig or hairpiece at a specialty shop just for cancer patients. Someone even may come to your home to help you. You also can buy a wig or hairpiece through a catalog or by phone. Call the American Cancer society for more information. (See page 50.)
- Consider borrowing a wig or hairpiece, rather than buying one. Check with the local chapter of the American Cancer Society or with the social work department at your hospital.
- Remember that a hairpiece needed because of cancer treatment is a tax-deductible expense and may be at least partially covered by your health insurance. Be sure to check your policy.

Losing hair from your head, face, or body can be hard to accept. It's common—and perfectly all right—to feel angry or depressed about this loss. Talking about your feelings can help.

Fatigue/Anemia

Chemotherapy can reduce the bone marrow's ability to make red blood cells, which carry oxygen to all parts of your body. When there are too few red blood cells, body tissues don't get enough oxygen to do their work. This condition is called anemia.

Anemia can make you feel very weak and tired. Other symptoms of anemia include dizziness, chills, or shortness of breath. Be sure to report any of these symptoms to your doctor.

Your doctor will check your **blood cell count** often during your treatment. If your red count falls too low, you may need a blood transfusion to increase the number of red blood cells in your body.

Here are some things you can do to help yourself feel better if you develop anemia:
- Get plenty of rest. Sleep more at night and take naps during the day if you can.
- Limit your activities: Do only the things that are most important to you.
- Don't be afraid to get help when you need it. Ask family and friends to pitch in with things like child care, shopping, housework, or driving.
- Eat a well balanced diet.
- When sitting or lying down, get up slowly. This will help prevent dizziness.

Infection

Chemotherapy can make you more likely to get infections. This happens because most anticancer drugs affect the bone marrow and decrease its ability to produce **white blood cells**, the cells that fight many types of infections. An infection can begin in almost any part of your body, including your mouth, skin, lungs, urinary tract, rectum, and reproductive tract.

Your doctor will check your blood cell count often while you are getting chemotherapy. Your doctor also may add **colony stimulating factors** to your treatment to keep your blood count from getting too far below normal. In spite of these extra steps, however, your white blood cell count still may drop. If this happens, your doctor may postpone your next treatment or give you a lower dose of drugs for a while.

When your white count is lower than normal, it is very important to try to prevent infections by taking the following steps:

- Wash your hands often during the day. Be sure to wash them extra well before you eat and before and after you use the bathroom.
- Clean your rectal area gently but thoroughly after each bowel movement. Ask your doctor or nurse for advice if the area becomes irritated or if you have hemorrhoids. Also, check with your doctor before using enemas or suppositories. (See page 26.)
- Stay away from people who have diseases you can catch, such as a cold, the flu, measles, or chickenpox. Also try to avoid crowds.
- Stay away from children who recently have received immunizations, such as vaccines for polio, measles, mumps and rubella (German measles).
- Don't cut or tear the cuticles of your nails.
- Be careful not to cut or nick yourself when using scissors, needles, or knives.
- Use an electric shaver instead of a razor to prevent breaks or cuts in your skin.
- Use a soft toothbrush that won't hurt your gums.
- Don't squeeze or scratch pimples.
- Take a warm (not hot) bath, shower, or sponge bath every day. Pat your skin dry using a light touch. Don't rub.

- Use lotion or oil to soften and heal your skin if it becomes dry and cracked.
- Clean cuts and scrapes right away with warm water, soap, and an antiseptic.
- Wear protective gloves when gardening or cleaning up after animals and others, especially small children.
- Do not get any immunization shots without checking first with your doctor to see if it's all right.

Most infections come from the bacteria normally found on the skin and in the intestines and genital tract. In some cases, the cause of an infection may not be known. When your white blood cell count is low, your body may not be able to fight off infections. So, even if you take extra care, you still may get an infection.

Be alert to the signals that you might have an infection and check your body regularly for its signs, paying special attention to your eyes, nose, mouth, and genital and rectal areas. The symptoms of infection include:
- Fever over 100 degrees F.
- Chills.
- Sweating.
- Loose bowels. (This also can be a side effect of chemotherapy.)
- A burning feeling when you urinate.
- A severe cough or sore throat.
- Unusual vaginal discharge or itching.
- Redness, swelling, or tenderness, especially around a wound, sore, pimple, or intravenous catheter site.

Report any signs of infection to your doctor right away. This is especially important when your white blood cell count is low. If you have a fever, don't use aspirin, acetaminophen, or any other medicine to bring your temperature down without first checking with your doctor.

Blood Clotting Problems

Anticancer drugs can affect the bone marrow's ability to make **platelets**, the blood cells that help stop bleeding by making your blood clot. If your blood does not have enough platelets, you may bleed or bruise more easily than usual, even from a minor injury.

Be sure to let your doctor know if you have unexpected bruising, small red spots under the skin, reddish or pinkish urine, or black or bloody bowel movements. Also report any bleeding from your gums or nose. Your doctor will check your platelet count often while you are having chemotherapy. If your platelet count falls too low, the doctor may give you a transfusion to build up the count.

Here are some ways to avoid problems if your platelet count is low:

• Don't take any medicine without first checking with your doctor or nurse. This includes aspirin or aspirin-free pain relievers, including acetaminophen, ibuprofen, and any other medicines you can buy without a prescription. These drugs may affect platelet function.

• Don't drink any alcoholic beverages unless your doctor says it's all right.

• Use a very soft toothbrush to clean your teeth.

• Clean your nose by blowing gently into a soft tissue.

• Take care not to cut or nick yourself when using scissors, needles, knives, or tools.

• Be careful not to burn yourself when ironing or cooking. Use a padded glove when you reach into the oven.

• Avoid contact sports and other activities that might result in injury.

Mouth, Gum, and Throat Problems

Good oral care is important during cancer treatment. Anticancer drugs can cause sores in the mouth and throat. They also can make these tissues dry and irritated or cause them to bleed. In addition to being painful, mouth sores can become infected by the many germs that live in the mouth. Because infections can be hard to fight during chemotherapy and can lead to serious problems, it's important to take every possible step to prevent them.

Here are some suggestions for keeping your mouth, gums, and throat healthy:

• If possible, see your dentist before you start chemotherapy to have your teeth cleaned and to take care of any problems such as cavities, abscesses, gum disease, or poorly fitting dentures. Ask your dentist to show you the best ways to brush and floss your teeth during chemotherapy. Chemotherapy can make you more likely to get cavities, so your dentist may suggest using a fluoride rinse or gel each day to help prevent decay.

- Brush your teeth and gums after every meal. Use a soft toothbrush and a gentle touch; brushing too hard can damage soft mouth tissues. Ask your doctor, nurse, or dentist to suggest a special type of toothbrush and/or toothpaste if your gums are very sensitive.
- Rinse your toothbrush well after each use and store it in a dry place.
- Avoid commercial mouthwashes that contain a large amount of salt or alcohol. Ask your doctor or nurse about a mild mouthwash that you might use.

If you develop sores in your mouth, be sure to contact your doctor or nurse because you may need medical treatment for the sores. If the sores are painful or keep you from eating, you also can try these ideas:

- Ask your doctor if there is anything you can apply directly to the sores. You also may ask your doctor to prescribe a medicine you can use to ease the pain.
- Eat foods cold or at room temperature. Hot and warm foods can irritate a tender mouth and throat.
- Choose soft, soothing foods, such as ice cream, milkshakes, baby food, soft fruits (bananas and applesauce), mashed potatoes, cooked cereals, soft-boiled or scrambled eggs, cottage cheese, macaroni and cheese, custards, puddings, and gelatin. You also can puree cooked foods in the blender to make them smoother and easier to eat.
- Avoid irritating, acidic foods, such as tomatoes, citrus fruit, and fruit juice (orange, grapefruit, and lemon); spicy or salty foods; and rough, coarse, or dry foods such as raw vegetables, granola, and toast.

If mouth dryness bothers you or makes it hard for you to eat, try these tips:

- Ask your doctor if you should use an artificial saliva product to moisten your mouth.
- Drink plenty of liquids.
- Suck on ice chips, popsicles, or sugarless hard candy. You can also chew sugarless gum.

- Moisten dry foods with butter, margarine, gravy, sauces, or broth.
- Dunk crisp, dry foods in mild liquids.
- Eat soft and loused foods like those listed above.
- Use lip balm if your lips become dry.

Diarrhea

When chemotherapy affects the cells lining the intestine, the result can be diarrhea (loose stools). If you have diarrhea that continues for more than 24 hours, or if you have pain and cramping along with the diarrhea, call your doctor. In severe cases, the doctor may prescribe an antidiarrheal medicine. However, you should not take any over-the-counter antidiarrheal medicines without asking your doctor first.

You also can try these ideas to help control diarrhea:
- Eat smaller amounts of food, but eat more often.
- Avoid high-fiber foods, which can lead to diarrhea and cramping. High-fiber foods include whole grain breads and cereals, raw vegetables, beans, nuts, seeds, popcorn, and fresh and dried fruit. Eat low fiber foods instead. Low-fiber foods include white bread, white rice or noodles, creamed cereals, ripe bananas, canned or cooked fruit without skins, cottage cheese, yogurt, eggs, mashed or baked potatoes without the skin, pureed vegetables, chicken or turkey without the skin, and fish.
- Avoid coffee, tea, alcohol, and sweets. Stay away from fried, greasy, or highly spiced foods, too. They are irritating and can cause diarrhea and cramping.
- Avoid milk and milk products if they make your diarrhea worse.
- Unless your doctor has told you otherwise, eat more potassium-rich foods because diarrhea can cause you to lose this important mineral. Bananas, oranges, potatoes, and peach and apricot nectars are good sources of potassium.
- Drink plenty of fluids to replace those you have lost through diarrhea. Mild, clear liquids, such as apple juice, water, weak tea, clear broth, or ginger ale, are best. Drink them slowly, and make sure they are at room temperatures. Let carbonated drinks lose their fizz before you drink them.
- If your diarrhea is severe, it is important to let your doc-

tor know. Ask your doctor if you should try a clear liquid diet to give your bowels time to rest. As you feel better, you gradually can add the low-fiber foods listed above. A clear liquid diet doesn't provide all the nutrients you need, so don't follow one for more than 3 to 5 days.

- If your diarrhea is very severe, you may need to get intravenous fluids to replace the water and nutrients you have lost.

Constipation

Some people who get chemotherapy become constipated because of the drugs they are taking. Others may become constipated because they are less active or less nourished than usual. Tell your doctor if you have not had a bowel movement for more than a day or two. You may need to take a laxative or stool softener or use an enema, but don't use these remedies unless you have checked with your doctor, especially if your white blood cell count is low.

You also can try these ideas to deal with constipation:

- Drink plenty of fluids to help loosen the bowels. Warm and hot fluids work especially well.
- Eat a lot of high-fiber foods. High-fiber foods include bran, wholewheat breads and cereals, raw or cooked vegetables, fresh and dried fruit, nuts, and popcorn.
- Get some exercise. Simply getting out for a walk can help, as can a more structured exercise program. Be sure to check with your doctor before becoming more active.

Nerve and Muscle Effects

Your nervous system affects just about all your body's organs and tissues. So it's not surprising that when chemotherapy affects the cells of the nervous system—as the drugs sometimes do—a wide range of side effects can result. For example, certain drugs can cause peripheral **neuropathy**, a condition that may make you feel a tingling, burning, weakness, or numbness in the hands and/or feet. Other nerve-related symptoms include loss of balance, clumsiness, difficulty picking up objects and buttoning clothing, walking problems, jaw pain, hearing loss, stomach pain, and constipation. In addition to affecting the nerves, certain anticancer drugs also can affect the muscles and make them weak, tired, or sore.

In some cases, nerve and muscle effects—though annoying—may not be serious. In other cases, nerve and muscle symptoms may indicate serious problems that need medical attention. Be sure to report any suspected nerve or muscle symptoms to your doctor.

Caution and common sense can help you deal with nerve and muscle problems. For example, if your fingers become numb, be very careful when grasping objects that are sharp, hot, or otherwise dangerous. If your sense of balance or muscle strength is affected, avoid falls by moving carefully, using handrails when going up or down stairs and using bath mats in the bathtub or shower. Do not wear slippery shoes.

Effects on Skin and Nails

You may have minor skin problems while you are having chemotherapy. Possible side effects include redness, itching, peeling, dryness, and acne. Your nails may become darkened, brittle, or cracked. They also may develop vertical lines or bands.

You will be able to take care of most of these problems yourself. If you develop acne, try to keep your face clean and dry and use over-the-counter medicated creams or soaps. For itching, apply cornstarch as you would a dusting powder. To help avoid dryness, take quick showers or sponge baths rather than long, hot baths. Apply cream and lotion while your skin is still moist and avoid perfume, cologne, or aftershave lotion that contains alcohol. You can strengthen your nails with the remedies sold for this purpose, but be alert to signs of a worsening problem because these products can be irritating to some people. Protect your nails by wearing gloves when washing dishes, gardening, or performing other work around the house. Get further advice from your doctor if these skin and nail problems don't respond to your efforts. Be sure to let your doctor know if you have redness, pain, or changes around the cuticles.

Certain anticancer drugs, when given intravenously, may produce a fairly dramatic darkening of the skin all along the vein. Some people use makeup to cover the area, but this can become difficult and time-consuming if several veins are affected, which sometimes happens. The darkened areas usually will fade on their own a few months after treatment ends.

Exposure to the sun may increase the effects some anticancer drugs have on your skin. Check with your doctor or nurse about using a sunscreen lotion with a skin protection factor of 15 to protect against the sun's effects. They may even suggest that you avoid being in direct sunlight or that you use a product, such as zinc oxide, that blocks the sun's rays completely. Long-sleeve cotton shirts, hats, and pants also will block the sun.

Some people who have had radiation therapy develop "radiation recall" during their chemotherapy. During or shortly after certain anticancer drugs are given, the skin over the area that was treated with radiation turns red—a shade anywhere from light to very bright—and may itch or burn. This reaction may last hours or even days. You can soothe the itching and burning by putting a cool, wet compress over the affected area. Radiation recall reactions should be reported to your doctor or nurse.

Most skin problems are not serious, but a few demand immediate attention. For example, certain drugs given intravenously can cause serious and permanent tissue damage if they leak out of the vein. Tell your doctor or nurse right away if you feel any burning or pain when you are getting IV drugs. These symptoms don't always mean there's a problem, but they always must be checked out at once.

You should also let your doctor or nurse know right away if you develop sudden or severe itching, if your skin breaks out in a rash or hives, or if you have wheezing or any other trouble breathing. These symptoms may mean you are having an allergic reaction that may need to be treated at once.

Kidney and Bladder Effects

Some anticancer drugs can irritate the bladder or cause temporary or permanent damage to the kidneys. Be sure to ask your doctor if your anticancer drugs are among the ones that have this effect, and notify the doctor if you have any symptoms that might indicate a problem. Signs to watch for include:
- Pain or burning when you urinate.
- Frequent urination.

- A feeling that you must urinate right away ("urgency").
- Reddish or bloody urine.
- Fever.
- Chills.

In general, it's a good idea to drink plenty of fluids to ensure good urine flow and help prevent problems; this is especially important if your drugs are among those that affect the kidney and bladder. Water, juice, coffee, tea, soup, soft drinks, broth, ice cream, soup, popsicles, and gelatin are all considered fluids. Your doctor will let you know if you must increase your fluid intake.

You also should be aware that some anticancer drugs cause the urine to change color (orange, red, or yellow) or to take on a strong or medicine-like odor. For a short time, the color and odor of semen may be affected as well. Check with your doctor to see if the drugs you are taking have this effect.

Flu-Like Syndrome

Some people report feeling as though they have the flu a few hours to a few days after chemotherapy. Flu-like symptoms—muscle aches, headache, tiredness, nausea, slight fever, chills, and poor appetite—may last from 1 to 3 days. These symptoms also can be caused by an infection or by the cancer itself, so it's important to check with your doctor if you have flu-like symptoms.

Fluid Retention

Your body may retain fluid when you are having chemotherapy. This may be due to hormonal changes from your therapy, to the effect of the drugs themselves, or to your cancer. Check with your doctor or nurse if you notice swelling or puffiness in your face, hands, feet, or abdomen. You may need to avoid table salt and foods with a high sodium content. If the problem is severe, your doctor may prescribe **diuretics**, medicine to help your body get rid of excess fluids. However, don't take any over-the-counter diuretics without asking your doctor first.

Sexual Effects: Physical and Psychological

Chemotherapy may—but does not always—affect sexual

organs and functioning in both men and women. The side effects that might occur depend on the drugs used and the person's age and general health.

Men: Chemotherapy drugs may lower the number of sperm cells, reduce their ability to move, or cause other abnormalities. These changes can result in infertility, which may be temporary or permanent. Infertility affects a man's ability to father a child but does not affect his ability to have sexual intercourse.

Because permanent sterility may occur, it's important to discuss this issue with your doctor before you begin chemotherapy. If you wish, you might consider sperm banking, a procedure that freezes sperm for future use.

Men undergoing chemotherapy should use an effective means of birth control with their partners during treatment because of the harmful effects of the drugs on chromosomes. Ask your doctor when you can stop using birth control for this purpose.

Women: Anticancer drugs can damage the ovaries and reduce the amount of hormones they produce. As a result, some women find that their menstrual periods become irregular or stop completely while they are having chemotherapy.

The hormonal effects of chemotherapy also may cause menopauselike symptoms such as hot flashes and itching, burning, or dryness of vaginal tissues. These tissue changes can make intercourse uncomfortable, but the symptoms often can be relieved by using a water-based vaginal lubricant. The tissue changes also can make a woman more likely to get vaginal infections. To help prevent infection, avoid oil-based lubricants such as petroleum jelly, wear cotton underwear and pantyhose with a ventilated cotton lining, and don't wear tight slacks or shorts. Your doctor also may prescribe a vaginal cream or suppository to reduce the chances of infection. If infection does occur, it should be treated right away. (See "Infection.")

Damage to the ovaries may result in infertility, the inability to become pregnant. In some cases, the infertility is a temporary condition; in other cases, it may be permanent. Whether infertility occurs, and how long it lasts, depends on many factors, including the type of drug, the dosage given, and the woman's age.

Although pregnancy may be possible during chemotherapy, it still is not advisable because some anticancer drugs may cause birth defects. Doctors advise women of childbearing age—from the teens through the end of menopause—to use birth control throughout their treatment.

If a woman is pregnant when her cancer is discovered, it may be possible to delay chemotherapy until after the baby is born. For a woman who needs treatment sooner, the doctor may suggest starting chemotherapy after the 12th week of pregnancy, when the fetus is beyond the stage of greatest risk. In some cases, termination of the pregnancy may be considered.

Sexuality: Sexual feelings and attitudes vary among people during chemotherapy. Some people find that they feel closer than ever to their partners and have an increased desire for sexual activity. Others experience little or no change in their sexual desire and energy level. Still others find that their sexual interest declines because of the physical and emotional stresses of having cancer and getting chemotherapy. These stresses may include worries about changes in appearance; anxiety about health, family, or finances; or side effects, including fatigue and hormonal changes.

A partner's concerns or fears also can affect the sexual relationship. Some may worry that physical intimacy will harm the person who has cancer; others may fear that they might "catch" the cancer or be affected by the drugs. Many of these issues can be cleared up by talking about misunderstandings. Both you and your partner should feel free to discuss sexual concerns with your doctor, nurse, or other counselor who can give you the information and the reassurance you need.

You and your partner also should try to share your feelings with one another. If it's difficult for you to talk to each other about sex, or cancer, or both, you may want to speak to a counselor who can help you communicate more openly. People who can help include psychiatrists, psychologists, social workers, marriage counselors, sex therapists, and members of the clergy.

If you were comfortable with and enjoyed sexual relations before starting therapy, chances are you will still find pleasure in physical intimacy during your treatment. You may discover, however, that intimacy takes on a new meaning and character. Hugging, touching, holding, and cuddling may become more important, while sexual intercourse may become less important. Remember that what was true before you started chemotherapy remains true now: There is no one "right" way to express your sexuality. It's up to you and your partner to determine together what is pleasurable and satisfying to you both.

The American Cancer Society has two free booklets on sexuality that may be helpful—one for women and one for men. Contact your local unit or the national office for copies.

EATING WELL DURING CHEMOTHERAPY

It is very important to eat as well as you can while you are undergoing treatment. People who eat well can cope with side effects better and are able to fight infection more easily. In addition, their bodies can rebuild healthy tissues faster.

Eating well during chemotherapy means choosing a balanced diet that contains all the nutrients the body needs. A good way to do this is to eat foods from each of the following food groups: fruits and vegetables; poultry, fish, and meat; cereals and breads; and dairy products. Eating well also means having a diet high enough in calories to keep your weight up and, most important, high enough in protein to build and repair skin, hair, muscles, and organs.

You also may need to drink extra amounts of fluid to protect your bladder and kidneys during your treatment. (See "Kidney and Bladder Effects.")

What If I Don't Feel Like Eating?

Even when you know it's important to eat well, there may be days when you feel you just can't. This may happen because side effects such as nausea or mouth and throat problems make it difficult or painful to eat. You also can lose your appetite if you feel depressed or tired. If this is the case, be sure to read the sections in this booklet on your particular discomforts. They will give you tips that can make it easier for you to eat.

When a poor appetite is the problem, try these hints:

• Eat small meals or snacks whenever you want. You don't have to eat three regular meals each day.

- Vary your diet and try new foods and recipes.
- When possible, take a walk before meals; this may make you feel hungrier.
- Try changing your mealtime routine. For example, eat by candlelight or in a different location.
- Eat with friends or family members. When eating alone, listen to the radio or watch TV.
- If you live alone, you might want to arrange for "Meals on Wheels" or a similar program to bring food to you. Ask your doctor, nurse, local American Cancer Society office, or the Cancer Information Service about these programs, which are provided in many communities.

The National Cancer Institute's booklet Eating Hints provides more tips about how to make eating easier and more enjoyable. It also gives many ideas about how to eat well and increase your protein and calorie intake during cancer treatment. For a free copy of Eating Hints, call the Cancer Information Service at 1-800-4-CANCER. (See "Resources.")

Can I Drink Alcoholic Beverages?

Small amounts of alcohol can help you relax and increase your appetite. On the other hand, alcohol may interact with some drugs to reduce their effectiveness or worsen their side effects. For this reason, some people must drink less alcohol or avoid alcohol completely during chemotherapy. Be sure to ask your doctor if it's okay for you to drink beer, wine, or other alcoholic beverages.

Should I Take Vitamin or Mineral Supplements?

There is no single answer to this question, but one thing is clear: No diet or nutritional plan can "cure" cancer, and taking vitamin and mineral supplements should never be considered a substitute for medical care. You should not take any supplements without your doctor's knowledge and consent.

TALKING WITH YOUR DOCTOR & NURSE

Some people with cancer want to know every detail about their condition and their treatment. Others prefer only general information. The choice of how much information to seek is yours, but there are questions that every person getting che-

motherapy should ask. These include:
- Why do I need chemotherapy?
- What are the benefits of chemotherapy?
- What are the risks of chemotherapy?
- What drug or drugs will I be taking?
- How will the drugs be given?
- Where will I get my treatments?
- How long will my treatment last?
- What are the possible side effects?
- Are there any side effects that I should report right away?
- Are there any other possible treatment methods for my type of cancer?

This list is just a start. You always should feel free to ask your doctor, nurse, and pharmacist as many questions as you want. If you don't understand their answers, keep asking until you do. Remember, when it comes to cancer and cancer treatment there is no such thing as a "stupid" question. To make sure you get all the answers you want, you may find it helpful to draw up a list of questions before your appointment. Some people even keep a "running list" and jot down each new question as it occurs to them.

To help remember your doctor's answers, you may want to take notes during your appointment. Don't feel shy about asking your doctor to slow down when you need more time to write. You might also ask if you can use a tape recorder during your visit. That way, you can review your conversation later as many times as you wish. Some doctors like this idea and others don't, so be sure to check before you try it. Another way to help you remember is to bring a friend or family member to sit with you while you talk to your doctor. This person can help you understand what your doctor says during your visit and help refresh your memory afterward.

CHEMOTHERAPY AND YOUR EMOTIONS

Chemotherapy can bring major changes to a person's life. It can affect overall health, threaten a sense of well-being, disrupt day-to-day schedules, and put a strain on personal relationships. No wonder, then, that many people feel fearful, anxious, angry, or depressed at some point during their chemotherapy.

These emotions are perfectly normal and understandable, but they also can be disturbing. Fortunately, there are ways to cope with these emotional "side effects," just as there are ways to cope with the physical side effects of chemotherapy.

How Can I Get the Support I Need?

There are many sources of support you can draw on. Here are some of the most important:

- Doctors and nurses. If you have questions or worries about your cancer treatment, talk with members of your health care team. (See "Talking With Your Doctor and Nurse.")
- Counseling professionals. There are many kinds of counselors who can help you express, understand, and cope with the emotions cancer treatment can cause. Depending on your preferences and needs, you might want to talk with a psychiatrist, psychologist, social worker, sex therapist, or member of the clergy.
- Friends and family members. Talking with friends or family members can help you feel a lot better. Often, they can comfort and reassure you in ways that no one else can. You may find, though, that you'll need to help them help you. At a time when you might expect that others will rush to your aid, you may have to make the first move.

Many people do not understand cancer, and they may withdraw from you because they're afraid of your illness. Others may worry that they will upset you by saying "the wrong thing."

You can help relieve these fears by being open in talking with others about your illness, your treatment, your needs, and your feelings. By talking openly, you can correct mistaken ideas about cancer. You can also let people know that there's no single "right" thing to say, so long as their caring comes through loud and clear. Once people know they can talk with you honestly, they may be more willing and able to open up and lend their support.

The National Cancer Institute's booklet *Taking Time* offers useful advice to help cancer patients and their families and friends communicate with one another. (See "Resources.")

- Support groups. Support groups are made up of people who are going through the same kinds of experiences as you. Many people with cancer find they can share thoughts and feelings with group members that they don't feel comfortable sharing with anyone else. Support groups also can serve as an important source of practical information about living with cancer.

Support can also be found in one-to-one programs that put you in touch with another person very similar to you in terms of age, sex, type of cancer, and so forth. In some programs, this person comes to visit you. In others, a "hotline" puts you in touch with someone you can talk with on the telephone.

Sources for information about support programs include your hospital's social work department, the local office of your American Cancer Society, and the National Cancer Institute's Cancer Information Service. (See "Resources.")

How Can I Make My Daily Life Easier?

Here are some tips to help yourself while you are getting chemotherapy:

- Try to keep your treatment goals in mind. This will help you keep a positive attitude on days when the going gets rough.
- Remember that eating well is very important. Your body needs food to rebuild tissues and regain strength.
- Learn as much as you want to know about your disease and its treatment. This can lessen your fear of the unknown and increase your feeling of control.
- Keep a journal or diary while you're in treatment. A record of your activities and thoughts can help you understand the feelings you have as you go through treatment, and highlight questions you need to ask your doctor or nurse. You also can use your journal to record the steps you take to cope with side effects and how well those steps work. That way, you'll know which methods worked best for you in case you have the same side effects again.
- Set realistic goals and don't be too hard on yourself. You may not have as much energy as usual, so try to get as much rest as you can, let the "small stuff" slide, and only do the things that are most important to you.
- Try new hobbies and learn new skills. Exercise if you can. Using your body can make you feel better about yourself, help you get rid of tension or anger, and build your appe-

tite. Ask your doctor or nurse about a safe and practical exercise program.

How Can I Relieve Stress?

You can use a number of methods to cope with the stresses of cancer and its treatment. The techniques described here can help you relax. Try some of these methods to find the one (or ones) that work best for you. You may want to check with your doctor before using these techniques, especially if you have lung problems.

- Muscle tension and release. Lie down in a quiet room. Take a slow, deep breath. As you breathe in, tense a particular muscle or group of muscles. For example, you can squeeze your eyes shut, frown, clench your teeth, make a fist, or stiffen your arms or legs. Hold your breath and keep your muscles tense for a second or two. Then breathe out, release the tension, and let your body relax completely. Repeat the process with another muscle or muscle group.

You also can try a variation of this method, called "progressive relaxation." Start with the toes of one foot and, working upward, progressively tense and relax all the muscles of one leg. Next, do the same with the other leg. Then tense and relax the rest of the muscle groups in your body, including those in your scalp. Remember to hold your breath while tensing your muscles and to breathe out when releasing the tension.

- Rhythmic breathing. Get into a comfortable position and relax all your muscles. If you keep your eyes open, focus on a distant object. If you close your eyes, imagine a peaceful scene or simply clear your mind and focus on your breathing.

Breathe in and out slowly and comfortably through your nose. If you like, you can keep the rhythm steady by saying to yourself, "In, one two; Out, one two." Feel yourself relax and go limp each time you breathe out.

You can do this technique for just a few seconds or for up to 10 minutes. End your rhythmic breathing by counting slowly and silently to three.

- Biofeedback. With training in biofeedback, you can control body functions such as heart rate, blood pressure, and muscle tension. A machine will sense when your body shows signs of tension and will let you know in some way such as making a sound or flashing a light. The machine will also give you feedback when you relax your body. Eventually, you will be able to control your relaxation responses without having to depend on feedback from the machine. Your doctor or nurse can refer you to someone trained in teaching biofeedback.

• Imagery. Imagery is a way of daydreaming that uses all your senses. It usually is done with your eyes closed. To begin, breathe slowly and feel yourself relax. Imagine a ball of healing energy— perhaps a white light—forming somewhere in your body. When you can "see" the ball of energy, imagine that as you breathe in you can blow the ball to any part of the body where you feel pain, tension, or discomfort such as nausea. When you breathe out, picture the air moving the ball away from your body, taking with it any painful or uncomfortable feelings. (Be sure to breathe naturally; don't blow.) Continue to picture the ball moving toward you and away from you each time you breathe in and out. You may see the ball getting bigger and bigger as it takes away more and more tension and discomfort.

To end the imagery, count slowly to three. breathe in deeply, open your eyes, and say to yourself, "I feel alert and relaxed."

If you choose to use imagery as a relaxation technique, please be sure to read the caution in the following section.

• Visualization. Visualization is a method that is similar to imagery. With visualization, you create an inner picture that represents your fight against cancer. Some people getting chemotherapy use images of rockets blasting away their cancer cells or of knights in armor battling their cancer cells. Others create an image of their white blood cells or their drugs attacking the cancer cells.

Visualization and imagery may help relieve stress and increase your sense of self-control. But it is very important to remember that they cannot take the place of the medical care your doctor prescribes to treat your cancer.

• Hypnosis. Hypnosis puts you in a trance-like state that can help reduce discomfort and anxiety. You can be hypnotized by a qualified person, or you can learn how to hypnotize yourself. If you are interested in learning more, ask your doctor or nurse to refer you to someone trained in the technique.

• Distraction. You use distraction any time an activity takes your mind off your worries or discomforts. Try watching TV, listening to the radio, reading, going to the movies, or working with your hands by doing needlework or puzzles, building models, or painting. You may be surprised how comfortably the time passes.

PAYING FOR CHEMOTHERAPY

The cost of chemotherapy varies with the kinds and dose of drugs used, how long and how often they are given, and whether you get them at home, in a clinic or office, or in the hospital. Most health insurance policies (including Medicare Part B. which helps pay for doctors' bills and many other medical services) cover at least part of the cost of many kinds of chemotherapy.

Sometimes, however, an insurer may not pay for the use of certain drugs for certain kinds of cancers— at least not at first. If your insurer denies payment for your treatment, don't give up. Most people do get payment eventually.

Teamwork with your doctor and the office staff is important. Be sure to let them know if you have been denied payment. They can consult with your insurer and help answer any questions your insurer may have. They also can consult with the company that makes the drug or drugs you are taking. Often, these companies can provide information or other services that will help you get payment.

In some states, Medicaid (which makes health care services available for people with financial need) may help pay for certain treatments. Contact the office that handles social services in your city or county to find out whether you are eligible for Medicaid and whether your chemotherapy is a covered expense.

If you need help paying for treatments, contact your hospital's social service office, the Cancer Information Service, or the local office of the American Cancer Society. (See "Resources.") They may be able to direct you to other sources of help. Another possibility is the Leukemia Society of America;

to find a chapter near you, check the white pages of your local telephone book.

A FINAL WORD

The National Cancer Institute hopes *Chemotherapy and You* helps you and your family, whether you are waiting to begin chemotherapy or already have begun your treatment. Discuss the information in this booklet with your doctor and nurse, and take good care of yourself during your chemotherapy. By working together, you, your family, and your health care providers will make the strongest possible team in your fight against cancer.

RESOURCES

Information about cancer is available from many sources, including the ones listed below. You may want to check for additional information at your local library or bookstore and from support groups in your community.

Cancer Information Service 1-800-4-CANCER

The Cancer Information Service, a program of the National Cancer Institute, is a nationwide telephone service for cancer patients and their families and friends, the public, and health care professionals. The staff can answer questions in English or Spanish and can send free National Cancer Institute booklets about cancer. They also know about local resources and services. One toll-tree number, 1-800-4CANCER (1-800-422-6237), connects callers with the office that serves their area.

PDQ

People who have cancer, those who care about them, and doctors need up-to-date and accurate information about cancer treatment. To meet these needs, PDQ was developed by NCI. PDQ contains an up-to-date list of clinical trails all over the country. The Cancer Information Service, at 1-800-4-CANCER, can provide PDQ information to doctors, patients, and the public.

American Cancer Society 1-800-ACS-2345

The American Cancer Society is a voluntary organization with a national office (at the above address) and local units all over the country. To obtain further information about services and activities in local areas, call the Society's toll-free number, 1-800-ACS-2345 (1-800-227-2345), or the number listed under American Cancer Society in the white pages of the telephone book.

Other Booklets

National Cancer Institute printed materials, including the booklets listed below, are available from the Cancer Information Service free of charge by calling 1-800-4-CANCER.
- Advanced Cancer: Living Each Day
- Eating Hints for Cancer Patients
- Facing Forward: A Guide for Cancer Survivors
- Questions and Answers About Pain Control (also available from the American Cancer Society)
- Radiation Therapy and You: A Guide to Self-Help During Treatment
- Taking Time: Support for People With Cancer and the People Who Care About Them
- What are Clinical Trials All About?
- What You Need To Know About Cancer. A series of booklets about different types of cancer.
- When Cancer Recurs: Meeting the Challenge Again

GLOSSARY

This glossary reviews the meaning of some words used in Chemotherapy *and You*. It also explains some words related to chemotherapy that are not mentioned in this booklet but that you may hear from your doctor or nurse.

Adjuvant therapy: Anticancer drugs or hormones given after surgery and/or radiation to help prevent the cancer from coming back.

Alopecia: Hair loss.

Anemia: Having too few red blood cells. Symptoms of anemia include feeling tired weak and short of breath.

Anorexia: Poor appetite.

Antiemetic: A medicine that prevents or controls nausea and vomiting.

Benign: A term used to describe a tumor that is not cancerous.

Biological therapy: Treatment to stimulate or restore the ability of the immune system to fight infection and disease. Also called immunotherapy.

Blood count: The number of red blood cells, white blood cells, and platelets in a sample of blood. This is also called complete blood count (CBC).

Bone marrow: The inner, spongy tissue of bones where blood cells are made.

Cancer: A general name for more than 100 diseases in which abnormal cells grow out of control; a malignant tumor.

Catheter: A thin flexible tube through which fluids can enter or leave the body.

Central venous catheter: A special thin, flexible tube placed in a large vein. It remains there for as long as it is needed to deliver and withdraw fluids.

Chemotherapy: The use of drugs to treat cancer.

Chromosomes: Threadlike bodies found in the nucleus, or center part, of a cell that carry the information of heredity.

Clinical trials: Medical research studies conducted with volunteers. Each study is designed to answer scientific questions and to find better ways to prevent or treat cancer.

Colony-stimulating factors: Substances that stimulate the production of blood cells. Treatment with colony-stimulating tractors (CSF) can help the blood-forming tissue recover from the effects of chemotherapy and radiation therapy. These include granulocyte colony-stimulating factors (G-CSF) and granulocytemacrophage colony-stimulating tractors (GM-CSF).

Combination chemotherapy: The use of more than one drug to treat cancer.

Diuretics: Drugs that help the body get rid of excess water and salt.

Gastrointestinal: Having to do with the digestive tract, which includes the mouth, esophagus, stomach, and intestines.

Hormones: Natural substances released by an organ that can influence the function of other organs in the body.
Infusion: Slow and/or prolonged intravenous delivery of a drug or fluids.
Injection: Using a syringe and needle to push fluids or drugs into the body; often called a "shot."
Intra-arterial (IA): Into an artery.
Intracavitary (IC): Into a cavity or space, specifically the abdomen, pelvis, or the chest.
Intralesional (IL): Into the cancerous area in the skin.
Intramuscular (IM): Into a muscle.
Intrathecal (IT): Into the spinal fluid.
Intravenous (IV): Into a vein.
Malignant: Used to describe a cancerous tumor.
Metastasis: When cancer cells break away from their original site and spread to other parts of the body.
Palliative care: Treatment to relieve, rather than cure, symptoms caused by cancer. Palliative care can help people live more comfortably.
Peripheral neuropathy: A condition of the nervous system that usually begins in the hands and/or feet with symptoms of numbness, tingling, burning and/or weakness. Can be caused by certain anticancer drugs.
Per os (PO): By mouth; orally.
Platelets: Special blood cells that help stop bleeding.
Port: A small plastic or metal container surgically placed under the skin and attached to a central venous catheter inside the body. Blood and fluids can enter or leave the body through the port using a special needle.
Radiation therapy: Cancer treatment with radiation (high-energy rays).
Red blood cells: Cells that supply oxygen to tissues throughout the body.
Remission: The partial or complete disappearance of signs and symptoms of disease.
Stomatitis: Sores on the lining of the mouth.
Subcutaneous (SQ or SC): Under the skin.
Tumor: An abnormal growth of cells or tissues. Tumors may be benign (noncancerous) or malignant (cancerous).
White blood cells: The blood cells that fight infection.

RADIATION THERAPY AND YOU
A GUIDE TO SELF-HELP
DURING TREATMENT

National Institutes of Health
National Cancer Institute

INTRODUCTION

This booklet is for you if you are receiving radiation therapy for cancer. Its main purpose is to help you know what to expect and how to care for yourself during your treatment. It describes external radiation therapy and brachytherapy using radiation implants, the two most common types of radiation therapy. Information is included on radiation therapy methods and the general effects of treatment. There are also some self-help "pointers" for specific side effects.

You may not want to read this whole booklet at one time. Flip through it, read the sections that are of interest to you right now, and look at the others as needled. Because your treatment will be planned specially for you and the type of cancer you have, some sections of the booklet will not apply to you.

Radiation therapy can vary among different doctors and hospitals. Therefore, your treatment program or the advice of your doctor (the radiation oncologist) may differ from what you read here. Be sure to ask questions and discuss your concerns with your doctor, nurse, or radiation therapist. Ask whether they have other booklets that also might help you.

You will find some helpful sections at the back of this booklet. The page labeled "Notes" can he used to write down questions to ask your doctor, nurse, or radiation therapist. Words that relate to radiation therapy and other aspects of cancer care appear in bold throughout this booklet: these words are defined in the "Glossary." Knowing the meanings of words can help you understand more about your illness and the roles of the people involved in your care. The "Resources" section tells you how to get more information about cancer and services for cancer patients from the National Cancer Institute and the American Cancer Society.

RADIATION IN CANCER TREATMENT

What Is Radiation Therapy?

Radiation is a special kind of energy carried by waves or a stream of particles. It can come from special machines or from radioactive substances. Many years ago doctors learned how to use this energy to see inside the body and find disease. You've probably seen a chest x-ray or x-ray pictures of your teeth or your bones. When radiation is used at high doses (many times those used for x-ray exams), it can be used to treat cancer and other illnesses. Special equipment is used to aim the radiation at tumors or areas of the body where there is disease. The use of high-energy rays or particles to treat disease is called radiation therapy. Sometimes it's called radiotherapy, x-ray therapy, cobalt therapy, electron beam therapy or irradiation.

How Does Radiation Therapy Work?

High doses of radiation can kill cells or keep them from growing and dividing. Radiation therapy is a useful tool for treating cancer because cancer cells grow and divide more rapidly than many of the normal cells around them. Although some normal cells are affected by radiation, most normal cells appear to recover more fully from the effects of radiation than do cancer cells. Doctors carefully limit the intensity of treatments and the area being treated so that the cancer will be affected more than normal tissue.

What Are the Benefits and Goals of Radiation Therapy?

Radiation therapy is an effective way to treat many kinds

of cancer in almost any part of the body. Half of all people with cancer are treated with radiation, and the number of cancer patients who have been cured is rising every day. For many patients, radiation is the only kind of treatment needed. Thousands of people are free of cancer after having radiation treatments alone or in combination with surgery, chemotherapy, or biological therapy.

Doctors can use radiation before surgery to shrink a tumor. After surgery, radiation therapy may be used to stop the growth of any cancer cells that remain. Your doctor may choose to use radiation therapy and surgery at the same time. This procedure, known as **intraoperative radiation**, is explained more fully on page 13. In some cases, doctors use radiation along with anticancer drugs to destroy the cancer, instead of surgery.

Even when curing the cancer is not possible, radiation therapy still can bring relief. Many patients find the quality of their lives improved when radiation therapy is used to shrink tumors and reduce pressure, bleeding, pain, or other symptoms of cancer. This is called **palliative care**.

Are There Risks Involved?

Like many other treatments for disease, there are risks for patients who are receiving radiation therapy. The brief high doses of radiation that damage or destroy cancer cells also can hurt normal cells. When this happens, the patient has side effects. These side effects and what to do about them are discussed later in this booklet. The risk of side effects is usually less than the benefits of killing cancer cells.

Your doctor will not advise you to have any treatment unless the benefits—control of disease and relief from symptoms—are greater than the known risks. Although it will be many years before scientists know all of the possible risks of radiation therapy, they now know that it can control cancer.

How is Radiation Therapy Given?

Radiation therapy can be in either of two forms: external or internal. Some patients have both forms, one after the other.

Most people who receive radiation therapy for cancer have the external type. It is usually given during outpatient visits to a hospital or treatment center. In external therapy, a machine directs the high-energy rays or particles at the cancer and the normal tissue surrounding it.

One type of machine that is used for radiation therapy is called a **linear accelerator**. High-energy rays may also come from a machine that contains a radioactive substance such as **cobalt-60**.

The various machines used for external radiation work in slightly different ways. Some are better for treating cancers near the skin surface; others work best on cancers deeper in the body. Your doctor decides which machine is best for you. External radiation is explained on page 9.

When **internal radiation** therapy is used, a radioactive substance, or source, is sealed in small containers such as thin wires or tubes called implants. The implant is placed directly into a tumor or inserted into a body cavity. Sometimes, after a tumor has been removed by surgery, implants are put into the area around the incision to kill any tumor cells that may remain.

Another type of internal radiation therapy uses unsealed radioactive sources. The source is either taken by mouth or is injected into the body. If you have this type of treatment, you will probably need to stay in the hospital for several days.

Who Gives Radiation Treatments?

A doctor who has had special training in using radiation to treat disease—**a radiation oncologist**—will prescribe the type and amount of treatment that best suits your needs. The radiation oncologist is the person referred to as "your doctor" throughout this booklet.

The radiation oncologist works closely with other doctors involved in your care and also heads a highly trained health care team. Your radiation therapy team may include:

• The **radiation physicist**, who makes sure that the equipment is working properly and ensures that the machines deliver the right dose of radiation.

• The **dosimetrist**, who helps carry out your treatment plan by calculating the number of treatments and how long each treatment should last.

• The radiation therapy nurse, who provides nursing care

and helps you learn about treatment and how to manage side effects.
• The **radiation therapist**, who sets you up for your treatments and runs the equipment that delivers the radiation.

You also may use the services of a **dietitian**, a **physical therapist**, a social worker, and other health care professionals.

Is Radiation Therapy Expensive?

Treatment of cancer with radiation can be costly. It requires very complex equipment and the services of many health care professionals. The exact cost of your radiation therapy will depend on the type and number of treatments you need.

Most health insurance policies, including Part B of Medicare, cover charges for radiation therapy. It's a good idea to talk with your doctor's office staff or the hospital business office about your policy and how expected costs will be paid.

In some states, the Medicaid program may help you pay for treatments. You can find out from the office that handles social services in your city or county whether you are eligible for Medicaid and whether your radiation therapy is a covered expense.

If you need financial aid, contact the hospital social service office, the Cancer Information Service, or the local office of the American Cancer Society. They may be able to direct you to sources of help. These organizations are listed in the "Resources" section.

EXTERNAL RADIATION THERAPY: WHAT TO EXPECT

How Does the Doctor Plan the Treatment?

The radiation used in radiation therapy can come from a variety of sources. Your doctor may choose to use **x-rays**, an **electron beam**, or cobalt-60 **gamma rays**. Choosing which type of radiation to use depends on what type of cancer you have and on how deep into your body the doctor wants the radiation to penetrate. High-energy radiation is used to treat many types of cancer. Low-energy x-rays are used to treat some kinds of skin diseases.

After a physical exam and a review of your medical history, the radiation oncologist may need to do some special planning to pinpoint the treatment area. In a process called **simulation**, you will be asked to lie very still on a table while the radiation therapist uses a special x-ray machine to define your **treatment port** or **field**. This is the exact place on your body where the treatment will be aimed. You may have more than one treatment port. Simulation may take from a half hour to about 2 hours.

The radiation therapist often will mark the treatment port on your skin with tiny dots of colored, semi-permanent ink to outline the treatment area. Be careful when you bathe because the marks must not be washed off until all of your treatment is over. If they start to fade, tell the therapist who will darken them so that they can be seen easily. Do not try to draw over faded lines at home unless they will be completely gone before your next visit. If you do replace the marks, be sure to tell the therapist at your next visit.

Using the information from the simulation, other tests, and your medical background, your doctor will meet with the radiation physicist and the dosimetrist. Your doctor then decides how much radiation is needed, how it will be delivered, and how many treatments you should have. This process often takes several days.

After you have started the treatments, your doctor will follow your progress, checking your response to treatment and your overall well-being at least once a week. The treatment plan may be revised by your doctor, if needed. It's very important that you have all of your scheduled treatments to get the most benefit from your therapy. Unnecessary delays can lessen the effectiveness of your radiation treatment.

How Long Does the Treatment Take?

Radiation therapy usually is given 5 days a week for 6 or 7 weeks. When radiation is used for palliative care, the course of treatment lasts for 2 to 3 weeks. These types of schedules, which use small amounts of daily radiation, rather than a few large doses, help protect normal body tissues in the treatment area. Weekend rest breaks allow normal cells to recover. The total dose of radiation and the number of treatments you need will depend on the size and location of your cancer, type of tumor, your general health, and any other treatments you're receiving.

What Happens During Each Treatment Visit?

Before your treatment is given, you may need to change into a hospital gown or robe. It's best to wear clothing that is easy to take off and put on again.

In the treatment room, the radiation therapist will use the marks on your skin to locate the treatment area. You will sit in a special chair or lie down on a treatment table. For each external radiation therapy session, you will be in the treatment room about 15 to 30 minutes, but you will be getting your dose of radiation for only about 1 to 5 minutes of that time. Receiving external radiation treatments is painless, just like having an x-ray taken.

The radiation therapist may put special shields (or blocks) between the machine and certain parts of your body to help protect normal tissues and organs. There might also be plastic or plaster forms to help you stay in exactly the right place. *You will need to remain very still during the treatment so that the radiation reaches only the area where it's needed and the same area is treated each time.* You don't have to hold your breath—just breathe normally.

The radiation therapist will leave the treatment room before the machine is turned on. The machine is controlled from a small area that is nearby. You will be watched on a television screen or through a window in the control room. Although you may feel alone, keep in mind that you can be seen and heard at all times by the therapist who can talk with you through a speaker.

The machines used for radiation treatments are very large, and they make noises as they move around to aim at the treatment area from different angles. Their size and motion may be frightening at first. Remember that the machines are being moved and controlled by your radiation therapist. They are checked constantly to be sure they're working right. If you are concerned about anything that happens in the treatment room, ask your therapist to explain.

You will not see or hear the radiation, and, most likely, you won't feel anything. If you do feel ill or very uncomfortable during the treatment, tell your therapist at once. The machine can he stopped at any time.

What Is Hyperfractionated Radiation Therapy?

Radiation is usually given once a day in a dose that is based on the type and location of the tumor. In **hyperfractionated radiation** therapy, the daily dose is divided into smaller doses that are given more than once a day. If more than one treatment is given per day to an area, the treatments usually are separated by 4 to 6 hours. Doctors are studying hyperfractionated therapy to see if it is equally or even more effective than once-a-day therapy. Early results in certain tumors are encouraging, and hyperfractionated therapy is becoming a more common way to give radiation treatments.

What Is Intraoperative Radiation?

Intraoperative radiation combines surgery and radiation therapy at the same time. The surgeon removes as much as possible of the tumor; then a large dose of radiation is given directly to the tumor bed and nearby areas where cancer cells might have spread. In some hospitals, there is an operating room right in the radiation therapy department; in others, the patient is treated in the radiation therapy department and then returned to the operating room for surgery. Sometimes high-dose intraoperative radiation is used in addition to external radiation therapy to give the cancer cells a larger amount of radiation than would be safe with external radiation alone.

What Are the Effects of Treatment?

External radiation therapy does not cause your body to become radioactive. There is no need to avoid being with other people because of your treatment. Even hugging, kissing, or having sexual relations with others poses no risk to them of radiation exposure.

Side effects of radiation therapy most often are related to the area that is being treated. Your doctor and nurse will tell you about the possible side effects and how you should deal with them. You should contact your doctor or nurse if you have any unusual symptoms during your treatment, such as coughing, sweating, fever, or unusual pain. Most side effects that occur during radiation therapy, although unpleasant, are not serious and can be controlled with medication or diet. They usually go away within a few weeks after treatment ends. However, some side effects can last longer. Many patients have no side effects at all. In another section of this booklet, "Managing Side Effects," you will find advice on how to cope with the side effects that might occur during and after your therapy.

Throughout your treatment, your radiation oncologist will regularly check on the effects of the treatment. You may not be aware of changes in the cancer, but you probably will notice decreases in pain, bleeding, or other discomforts you may have had, especially after your treatment is completed. You may continue to notice more improvements with time. Your doctor probably will recommend some tests to be sure that the radiation is causing as little damage to normal cells as possible. You may have routine blood tests to check the levels of **white blood cells** and **platelets**, which may be lower than normal during treatment.

What Can I Do to Take Care of Myself During Therapy?

Each patient's body responds to radiation therapy in its own way. That's why the doctor must plan, and sometimes adjust, your treatment just for you. In addition, your doctor or nurse will give you advice for caring for yourself at home that is specific for your treatment and the side effects that might result.

Nearly all cancer patients receiving radiation therapy need to take special care of themselves to protect their health and help the treatment succeed. Some guidelines to remember are given below:

- Be sure to get plenty of rest. Sleep as often as you feel the need. Your body will use a lot of extra energy over the course of your treatment, and you may feel very tired. In fact, fatigue may last for 4 to 6 weeks after your treatment is finished.
- Good nutrition is a must. Try to eat a balanced diet that will prevent weight loss. For patients who have problems with

eating or diet planning, the section titled "Managing Side Effects" offers practical tips.
- Avoid wearing tight clothes such as girdles or close-fitting collars over the treatment area. It's best to wear older garments that feel comfortable and that you can wash or throw away if the ink marks rub off on them.
- Be *extra* kind to the skin in the treatment area.
- Do not use any soaps, lotions, deodorants, medicines, perfumes, cosmetics, talcum powder, or other substances in the treated area without talking with your doctor.
- Wear loose, soft cotton clothing over the treated area.
- Do not starch your clothes.
- Do not rub or scrub treated skin.
- Do not use adhesive tape on treated skin. If bandaging is necessary, use paper tape. Try to apply the tape outside of the treatment area.
- Do not apply heat or cold (heating pad, ice pack, etc.) to the treatment area. Even hot water can hurt your skin, so use only lukewarm water for bathing the treated area.
- Use an electric shaver if you must shave the area—but only after checking with your doctor or nurse. Do not use a pre-shave lotion or hair remover products.
- Protect the area from the sun. If possible, cover treated skin with light clothing before going outside. Ask your doctor if you should use a lotion that contains a sunblock. If so, use a PABA sunscreen or a sunblocking product with a protection factor of at least 15. Reapply the sunscreen often, even after your skin has healed following your treatment. Continue to protect your skin from sunlight for at least 1 year after radiation therapy.
- Be sure your doctor knows about any medicines you are taking before starting treatment. If you need to start taking any medicines, even aspirin, let your doctor know before you start.
- Ask your doctor, nurse, or radiation therapist any questions you have. They are the only ones who can properly advise you about your treatment, side effects, at-home care, and any other medical concerns you may have.

INTERNAL RADIATION THERAPY: WHAT TO EXPECT

When Is Internal Radiation Therapy Used?

Your doctor may decide that very intense radiation given to a small area of your body is the best way to treat your cancer. Internal radiation therapy places the source of the high-energy rays as close as possible to the cancer cells so that fewer normal cells are exposed to radiation. By using internal radiation therapy, the doctor can give a higher total dose of radiation in a shorter time than is possible with external treatment. Instead of using a large radiation machine, the radioactive material is placed directly into (or as close as possible to) the affected area. Some of the radioactive substances used for internal radiation treatment include radium, cesium, iridium, iodine, phosphorus, and palladium.

Internal radiation therapy often is used for cancers of the head and neck, breast, uterus, thyroid, cervix, and prostate. Your doctor may recommend a combination of internal and external radiation therapy.

Implant radiation as used in this booklet means internal radiation treatment. You also may hear the terms **interstitial radiation, intracavitary radiation,** or **brachytherapy**; each is a form of internal radiation therapy. Some people use the term "brachytherapy" whenever they are talking about any form of internal radiation therapy.

When interstitial radiation is given, the radiation source is placed right in the affected tissue, usually in small tubes or containers. These **implants** may be temporary or permanent. When intracavitary radiation is used, a container of radioactive material is placed in a cavity of the body such as the uterus. In brachytherapy, the radioactive source, which is sealed in a small container, is placed on the surface of the body near the tumor or a short distance from the affected area. The radioactive source also may be delivered to the tumor through tubes; this is called **remote brachytherapy.** Internal radiation also may be given by injecting a solution of radioactive substance into the bloodstream or a body cavity. When the substance is injected, it is not sealed in a container and may be called **unsealed internal radiation therapy.**

How Is the Implant Placed in the Body?

For most types of implants, you will need to be in the hospital and have general or local anesthesia while the doctor places the container for the radioactive material in your body. In many hospitals, the radioactive material is placed in the container after you return to your room so that others are not exposed to radiation.

To get the radiation as close as possible to the cancer, doctors may use implants of radioactive material sealed in wires, seeds, capsules, or needles. The type of implant and the method of placing it depend on the size and location of the cancer. Implants may be put right into the tumor, in special applicators inside a body cavity, on the surface of a tumor, or in the area from which the tumor has been taken.

Does the Implant Spread Radiation to Others?

The radioactive substance in your implant may transmit rays outside your body. While you're receiving implant therapy, the hospital may require you to stay in a private room. Although the nurses and other people caring for you will not be able to spend a long time in your room, they will give you all of the care you need. You should call for a nurse when you need one, but keep in mind that the nurse will work quickly and speak to you from the doorway more often than from your bedside. In most cases, your urine and stool will contain no radioactivity. However, either one may contain some radioactive material if you have unsealed internal radiation therapy.

There also will be limits on visitors while your implant is in place. Most hospitals do not let children younger than 18 or pregnant women visit patients who have an implant. Visitors should sit at least 6 feet from your bed and stay for only a short time each day (10 to 30 minutes). Have visitors ask your nurse for specific instructions before they enter your room.

Are There Any Side Effects?

You are not likely to have severe pain or feel ill during implant therapy. However, if an applicator is holding your implant in place, it may be somewhat uncomfortable. If you need it, the doctor will order medicine to help you relax or to relieve pain. Some patients feel drowsy, weak, or nauseated after having the anesthesia to place the implant, but these effects do not last long.

Be sure to tell the nurse if you have any side effects such as burning, sweating, or other unusual symptoms. In the section of this booklet called "Managing Side Effects," you will find tips on skin care and what you can do about problems that might occur after implant therapy.

How Long Does the Implant Stay in Place?

The total amount of time that an implant is left in place depends on the dose (amount) of radioactivity with which the patient is treated. The implant may be low dose rate and left in place for several days, or it may be high dose rate and removed after a few minutes. Generally, low dose rate implants are left in place from 1 to 7 days. Your treatment schedule will depend on the type of cancer, where it is, your general health, and other cancer treatments you have had. Depending on where the implant is placed, you may have to stay in bed and lie fairly still to keep the implant from shifting.

For some cancer sites, the implant may be left in place permanently. If your implant is permanent, you may need to stay in your room away from other people in the hospital for a few days while the radiation is most active. The implant will lose energy each day, so by the time you are ready to go home, the radiation in your body will be much weaker. Your doctor will advise you if there are any special precautions you need to use at home.

High dose rate remote brachytherapy allows a person to be treated within a few minutes in inpatient or outpatient clinics. With remote brachytherapy, a very powerful radioactive source travels by remote control through tubes, or **catheters**, to the tumor. The radioactivity remains at the tumor for only a few minutes. This procedure is done by the brachytherapy team, who will watch you on a closed-circuit television. They will talk to you through an intercom In some cases, several remote treatments may be required. Sometimes, the catheter stays in place between treatments and sometimes it is removed, depending on your condition.

High dose rate treatments are short (usually a few minutes) and result in less discomfort than other types of radiation therapy. Because radioactive materials are not left in your body, you can return home soon after you recover. Remote brachytherapy has been used to treat cancers of the cervix, breast, lung, pancreas, prostate, and esophagus.

What Happens After the Implant Is Removed?

Usually there is no need to have an anesthetic to take out the implant. Most can be taken out right in the patients hospital room. If you had to stay in bed during implant therapy, you might have to remain in the hospital an extra day or so after the implant is removed. Once the implant is removed, there is no radioactivity in your body. The nurses and your visitors no longer will have to observe any special rules.

Your doctor will tell you if you should limit your activities after leaving the hospital. Most patients are allowed to do as much as they feel like doing. You may need some extra sleep or rest breaks during your first days at home, but you will feel stronger quickly.

The area that has been treated with an implant may be sore or sensitive for some time after therapy. Your doctor may advise you to limit sports and sexual activity for a while if they cause irritation in the treatment area.

MANAGING SIDE EFFECTS

Are Side Effects the Same for Everyone?

The side effects of radiation treatment vary from patient to patient. You may have no side effects or only a few mild ones through your course of treatment. Or you may have more serious side effects. The side effects that you have depend mostly on the treatment dose and the part of your body that is treated. Your general health also can affect how your body reacts to radiation therapy and whether you have side effects. Before beginning your treatment, ask your doctor and nurse about the side effects you might experience, how long they might last, and how serious they might be.

There are two main types of side effects: acute and chronic.

Acute, or short-term, side effects occur close to the time of the treatment and usually are gone completely within a few weeks of finishing therapy. Chronic, or long-term, side effects may take months or years to develop and usually are permanent.

The most common side effects are fatigue, skin changes, and loss of appetite. They can result from radiation to any treatment site. Other side effects are related to treatment of specific areas. For example, temporary or permanent hair loss may be a side effect of radiation treatment to the head. This chapter discusses common side effects first. Then side effects involving specific body parts are described.

Fortunately, most side effects will go away in time. In the meantime, there are ways to reduce the discomfort they cause. If you have a side effect that is particularly severe, the doctor may prescribe a break in your treatments or change the kind of treatment you're receiving.

Be sure to tell your doctor, nurse, or radiation therapist about any side effects that you notice. They can help you treat the problems and tell you how to lessen the chances that the side effects will come back. The information in this booklet can serve as a guide to handling some side effects, but it cannot replace talking with your health care team.

Will Side Effects Limit My Activity?

Not necessarily. It will depend on what side effects you have and how severe they are. Many patients are able to go to work, keep house, and enjoy leisure activities while they are receiving radiation therapy. Others find that they need more rest than usual and therefore cannot do as much. You should try to do the things you enjoy as long as you don't become too tired.

Your doctor may suggest that you limit activities that might irritate the area being treated. In most cases, you can have sexual relations if you wish. Your desire for physical intimacy may be lower because radiation therapy may cause you to feel more tired than usual. For most patients, these feelings are temporary.

What Causes Fatigue

During radiation therapy, the body uses a lot of energy

healing itself. Stress related to your illness, daily trips for treatment, and the effects of radiation on normal cells all may contribute to fatigue. Most people begin to feel tired after a few weeks of radiation therapy. Feelings of weakness or weariness will go away gradually after your treatment is finished.

You can help yourself during radiation therapy by not trying to do too much. If you feel tired, limit your activities and use your leisure time in a restful way. Do not feel that you have to do all the things you normally do. Try to get more sleep at night, and rest during the day if you can.

If you have been working a full-time job, you may want to continue. Although treatment visits are time-consuming, you can ask your doctor's office or the radiation therapy department to help by trying to schedule treatments with your workday in mind.

Some patients prefer to take a few weeks off from work while they're receiving radiation therapy; others work a reduced number of hours. You may want to speak frankly with your employer about your needs and wishes during this time. You may be able to agree on a part-time schedule, or perhaps you can do some work at home.

Whether you're going to work or not, it's a good idea to ask family members or friends to help with daily chores, shopping, child care, housework, or driving. Neighbors may be able to help by picking up groceries for you when they do their own shopping. You also could ask someone to drive you to and from your treatment visits to help conserve your energy.

How Are Skin Problems Treated?

You may notice that your skin in the treatment area may begin to look reddened, irritated, sunburned, or tanned. After a few weeks you may have very dry skin from the therapy. Ask your doctor or nurse for advice on relieving itching or discomfort. With some kinds of radiation therapy, treated skin may develop a "moist reaction," especially in areas where there are skin folds. When this happens, the skin is wet and it may become very sore. It's important to notify your doctor or nurse if your skin develops a moist reaction. They can give you some suggestions on how you can keep these areas dry. Other helpful tips can be found below.

During radiation therapy you will need to be very gentle with the skin in the treatment area. Avoid irritating treated skin. When you wash, use only lukewarm water and mild soap. Don't wear tight clothing over the area. It's important not to rub, scrub, or scratch any sensitive spots. Also avoid putting anything that is very hot or very cold, such as heating pads or ice packs, on your treated skin. Don't use any powders, creams, perfumes, deodorants, body oils, ointments, lotions, or home remedies in the treatment area while you're being treated or for several weeks afterward (unless approved by your doctor or nurse). Many skin products can leave a coating on the skin that can interfere with radiation therapy or healing.

Avoid exposing the area to the sun during treatment and for at least 1 year after your treatment is completed. If you expect to be in the sun for more than a few minutes you will need to be very careful. Wear protective clothing (such as a hat with a broad brim and a shirt with long sleeves) and use a sunscreen. Ask your doctor or nurse about using sunblocking lotions.

The majority of skin reactions to radiation therapy should go away a few weeks after treatment is finished. In some cases, though, the treated skin will remain darker than it was before.

What Can Be Done About Hair Loss?

Radiation therapy can cause hair loss, also known as **alopecia**, but only in the area being treated. For example, if you are receiving treatment to your hip, you will not lose the hair from your head. However, radiation to your head may cause you to lose some or all of the hair on your scalp. Many patients find that their hair grows back again after the treatments are finished, but accepting the loss of hair—whether from scalp, face, or body—can be a hard adjustment. The amount of hair that grows back will depend on how much radiation you receive and the type of radiation treatment your doctor recommends. Other types of treatment, such as chemotherapy, also can affect how your hair grows back. For example, if your radiation therapy is for palliative care, your hair probably will grow back slowly. However, if the goal of your radiation therapy is to cure rather than to relieve the symptoms of your cancer, then your hair may not grow back, and if it does, it probably will be very fine.

Although your scalp may be tender after the hair is lost, you may want to cover your head with a hat, turban, or scarf while you're in treatment. Also, you should wear a protective cap or scarf when you're in the sun. If you prefer a wig or toupee, be sure the lining does not irritate your scalp. A hairpiece that you need because of cancer treatment is a tax-deductible expense and may be covered in part by your health insurance. If you plan to buy a wig, it's a good idea to select it early in your treatment so that you can match the color and style to your own hair.

What About Side Effects on the Blood?

Sometimes radiation therapy can cause low white blood cell counts or low levels of platelets. These blood cells help your body fight infection and prevent bleeding. If your blood tests show this side effect, your treatment might be delayed for about a week to allow your blood counts to increase.

What If There Are Eating Problems?

Many side effects can cause problems with eating and digesting food, but you always should try to eat enough to help damaged tissues rebuild themselves. It's very important not to lose weight during radiation therapy. Try to eat small meals often and eat a variety of different foods. Your doctor or nurse can tell you whether your treatment calls for a special diet, and a dietitian will have a lot of ideas to help you maintain your weight.

Coping with short-term diet problems may be easier than you expect. There are a number of diet guides and recipe booklets for patients who need help with eating problems. Another NCI booklet, *Eating Hints*, tells how to get more calories and protein without eating more food and provides further tips to help you enjoy eating. The recipes it contains can be used for the whole family and are marked for people with special concerns, such as low-salt diets. (See Resources.)

If you have pain when you chew and swallow, your doctor may advise you to use a powdered or liquid diet supplement. Many of these products, available at the drugstore without prescription, are made in a variety of flavors. They are tasty when used alone, or they can be combined with other foods, such as pureed fruit, or added to milkshakes. Some of the companies that make diet supplements have produced recipe booklets to help you increase your nutrient intake. Ask your dietitian or pharmacist for further information.

You may lose interest in food during your treatment. Loss of appetite can happen when changes occur in normal cells. Some people just don't feel like eating because of stress from their illness and treatment or because the treatment changes the way foods taste. Even if you're not very hungry, it's important that you make every effort to keep your protein and calorie intake high. Doctors have found that patients who eat well can better handle both their cancer and the side effects of treatment.

The list below suggests ways to perk up your appetite when it's poor and to make the most of it when you do feel like eating.

- Eat when you are hungry, even if it is not mealtime.
- Eat several small meals during the day rather than three large ones.
- Use soft lighting, quiet music, brightly colored table settings, or whatever helps you feel good while eating.
- Vary your diet and try new recipes.
- If you enjoy company while eating, try to have meals with family or friends, or turn on the radio or television .
- Ask your doctor or nurse whether you can have a glass of wine or beer with your meal to increase your appetite. Keep in mind that in some cases, alcohol may not be allowed because of the chance that it will worsen the side effects of treatment. This may be especially true if you are receiving radiation therapy for cancer of the head or neck. (See information on effects to the mouth and throat.)
- When you feel up to it, make some simple meals in batches and freeze them to use later.
- Keep healthy snacks close by for nibbling when you get the urge.
- If other people offer to cook for you, let them. And don't be shy about telling them what you'd like to eat.
- If you live alone, you might want to arrange for "Meals

on Wheels" to bring food to you. Ask your doctor, nurse, local American Cancer Society office, or Cancer Information Service about "Meals on Wheels." This service is active in most large communities.

If you are able to eat only small amounts of food, you can increase the calories per serving by trying the following ideas:
- Add butter or margarine if you like the flavor.
- Mix canned cream soups with milk or half-and-half rather than water.
- Drink eggnogs, milkshakes, or prepared liquid supplements between meals.
- Add cream sauce or melted cheese to your favorite vegetables.

Some people find they can handle large amounts of liquids even when they don't feel like eating solid foods. If this is the case for you, try to get the most from each glassful by having drinks enriched with powdered milk, yogurt, honey, or prepared liquid supplements.

Does Radiation Therapy Affect the Emotions?

Nearly all patients who receive treatment for cancer feel some degree of emotional upset. It's not unusual to feel depressed, afraid, angry, frustrated, alone, or helpless. Radiation therapy may affect the emotions indirectly through fatigue or changes in hormone balance, but the treatment itself is not a direct cause of mental distress.

Many patients help themselves by talking about their feelings with a close friend, family member, chaplain, nurse, social worker, or psychologist with whom they feel at ease. You may want to ask your doctor or nurse about meditation or relaxation exercises that could help you unwind and feel better.

American Cancer Society nationwide programs can provide support. Groups such as the United Ostomy Association and the Lost Chord Club offer opportunities to meet with others who share the same problems and concerns. Some medical centers have formed peer support groups so that patients can meet to discuss their feelings and inspire each other.

There are several helpful books and other materials on this subject. The Cancer Information Service can direct you to reading matter and other resources in your area. (See Resources.)

What Side Effects Occur With Radiation Therapy to the Head and Neck Area?

Some people who are having radiation to the head and neck have redness and irritation in the mouth, a dry mouth, difficulty in swallowing, changes in taste, or nausea. Try not to let these symptoms keep you from eating.

Other problems that may occur during treatment to the head and neck are a loss of your sense of taste, earaches (caused by hardening of ear wax), and swelling or drooping of skin under the chin. There may be changes in your skin texture. You also may notice that your jaw feels stiff and that you cannot open your mouth as wide as before your treatment. Jaw exercises may help this problem. Report any side effects to your doctor or nurse and ask what you should do about them.

If you are receiving radiation therapy to the head or neck, you need to take especially good care of your teeth, gums, mouth, and throat. Side effects from treatment to these areas most often involve the mouth, which may be sore and dry.

Here are a few tips that may help you manage mouth problems:

- Avoid spices and coarse foods such as raw vegetables, dry crackers, and nuts.
- Don't smoke, chew tobacco, or drink alcohol.
- Stay away from sugary snacks that promote tooth decay.
- Clean your mouth and teeth often, using the method your dentist or doctor recommends.
- Do not use a commercial mouthwash; the alcohol content has a drying effect on mouth tissues.

Dental Care

Radiation treatment for head and neck cancer can increase your chances of getting cavities. Mouth care designed to prevent problems will be a very important part of your treatment. Before starting radiation therapy, notify your dentist and arrange for a complete dental/oral checkup. *Ask your dentist to consult with your radiation oncologist about any dental work you need before your radiation treatments begin.*

Your dentist probably will want to see you often over the course of your radiation therapy. Your dentist can give you very detailed instructions about caring for your mouth and

teeth to reduce the risk of tooth decay and will help you deal with possible problems such as soreness of the tissues in your mouth. It is important to your total well-being that you follow the dentist's advice while you're receiving radiation therapy. Most likely, you will be advised to:
- Clean teeth and gums thoroughly with a soft brush after meals and at least once more each day.
- Use a fluoride toothpaste that contains no abrasives.
- Floss gently between teeth daily, especially if you flossed regularly before your illness.
- Use a disclosing solution or tablet after brushing to reveal plaque that you've missed.
- Rinse your mouth well with a salt and baking soda solution after you brush. Use 1/2 teaspoon of salt and 1/2 teaspoon of baking soda in 1 quart of water.
- Apply **fluoride** regularly as prescribed by your dentist.

Your dentist can explain how to use disclosing tablets, how to mix the salt and baking soda mouthwash, and how to use the fluoride treatment method that best suits your needs. Most likely you can get printed instructions for proper dental care at the dentist's office.

Handling Mouth or Throat Problems

Soreness in your mouth or throat may appear in the second or third week of external radiation therapy. It is likely to decrease from the fifth week on and end a month or so after your treatment ends. You may have trouble swallowing during this time because your mouth feels dry. Your doctor or dentist can prescribe medicine for mouth discomfort and advise you about methods to relieve other mouth problems.

If you wear dentures you may notice that they no longer fit well. This may happen if the radiation causes swelling in your gums. It's important not to let your dentures cause gum sores that may become infected. You may need to stop wearing your dentures until your radiation therapy is over.

Your glands may produce less saliva than usual, making your mouth feel dry. It's helpful to sip cool drinks often throughout the day. Water probably is your best choice. In the morning, fill up a large cup or glass with ice, add water, and carry it with you so you have something to drink during the day. Keep a glass of cool water at your bedside at night, too. Many radiation therapy patients say that drinking carbonated beverages helps relieve dry mouth. Sugar-free candy or gum also may help. Avoid tobacco and alcoholic drinks because they will dry and irritate your mouth tissues even more. Moisten food with gravies and sauces to make eating easier. If these measures are not enough, ask your dentist about artificial saliva. Dry mouth may continue to be a problem even after treatment is over.

Tips on Eating

If you are having radiation therapy to the chest, you may find swallowing difficult or painful. Some patients say that it feels like something is stuck in their throat.

Soreness or dryness in your mouth or throat can make it hard to eat. However, there are several ways to ease your discomfort:

- Choose foods that taste good to you and are easy to eat.
- Try changing the consistency of foods by adding fluids and using sauces and gravies to make them softer.
- Avoid highly spiced foods and textures that are dry and rough such as crackers.
- Eat small meals and eat more frequently than usual.
- Cut your food into small, bite-sized pieces.
- Ask your doctor for special liquid medicines that can help you eat and swallow more easily by reducing the pain in your throat.
- Ask your doctor about liquid food supplements. These can help you meet your energy needs.
- If you are being treated for lung cancer and you get your doctors okay try to drink extra fluids. This will help keep mucus and other secretions thin and manageable.
- If your sense of taste changes during radiation therapy try different methods of food preparation.

Also many helpful suggestions can be found in the NCI booklet *Eating Hints*. (See Resources.)

What Side Effects Occur With Radiation Therapy to the Breast and Chest?

Radiation treatment to the chest may cause several changes.

You will notice some of these changes yourself and your treatment team will keep an eye on these and others. For example you may find that it is hard to swallow or that swallowing hurts. You may develop a cough. Or you may develop a fever notice a change in the color or amount of mucus when you cough or feel short of breath. It is important to let your treatment team know right away if you have any of these symptoms. Your doctor also may check your blood counts regularly especially if the radiation treatment area on your body is large. Just keep in mind that your doctor and nurse will be alert for these changes and will help you deal with them.

If you are receiving radiation therapy after a lumpectomy or mastectomy it's a good idea to go without wearing a bra whenever possible. If this is not possible, wear a soft cotton bra without underwires. This will help reduce the irritation to your skin in the treatment area. You may have several other side effects if you are receiving radiation therapy for breast cancer. For example, you may notice a lump in your throat or develop a dry cough. Or, your shoulder may feel stiff; if so, ask your doctor or nurse about exercises to keep your arm moving freely. Other side effects that may appear are breast soreness and swelling from fluid buildup in the treated area. These side effects, as well as skin reddening or tanning, most likely will disappear in 4 to 6 weeks. If fluid buildup continues to be a problem, your doctor will tell you what steps to take.

Women who have radiation therapy after a lumpectomy may notice other changes in the breast after the therapy. These long-term side effects may continue for a year or longer after treatment. The redness of the skin will fade, and you may notice that your skin is slightly darker, just as when a sunburn fades to a suntan. The pores may be enlarged and more noticeable. Some women report increased sensitivity of the skin on the breast; others have decreased feeling. The skin and the fatty tissue of the breast may feel thicker, and you may notice that your breast is firmer than it was before your radiation treatment. Sometimes the size of your breast changes—it may become larger because of fluid buildup or smaller because of the development of fibrous tissue. Many women have little or no change in size.

Your radiation therapy plan may include implants of radioactive material a week or two after external treatment is completed. You may have some breast tenderness or a feeling of tightness while the implants are in your breast. After they are removed, you are likely to notice some of the same effects that occur with external treatment. If so, follow the advice given above and let your doctor know about any problems that persist.

After 10 to 12 months, no further changes are likely to be caused by the radiation therapy. If you see new changes in breast size, shape, appearance, or texture after this time, report them to your doctor at once.

What Side Effects Occur with Radiation Therapy to the Stomach and Abdomen?

If you are having radiation treatment to the stomach or some portion of the abdomen, you may have to deal with an upset stomach, nausea, or diarrhea. Your doctor can prescribe medicines to relieve these problems. Do not take any home remedies during your treatment unless you first check with your doctor or nurse.

Managing Nausea

Some patients report feeling queasy for a few hours right after radiation therapy to the stomach or abdomen. If you have this problem, do not eat for several hours before your treatment time. You may be able to handle the treatment better on an empty stomach. After your treatment, you may find it helpful to wait 1 to 2 hours before eating again. If the problem persists, ask your doctor to prescribe a medicine (an **antiemetic**) to prevent nausea. If antiemetics are prescribed, try to take them when your doctor suggests, even if you sometimes feel that they are not needed.

If your stomach feels upset just before your treatment, try a bland snack such as toast or crackers and apple juice before your appointment. This type of side effect may be related to your emotions and concerns about treatment. Try to unwind a bit before you have your treatment. If you have to spend time in a waiting room, reading a book, writing letters, or working a crossword puzzle may help you relax.

Here are some tips to help an unsettled stomach:
- Stick to any special diet that your doctor or dietitian gives you.
- Eat small meals.
- Eat often and try to eat and drink slowly.
- Avoid foods that are fried or are high in fat.
- Drink cool liquids between meals.
- Eat foods that have only a mild aroma and those that can be served cool or at room temperature.
- For a severe upset stomach, try a clear liquid diet (broth and juices) or bland foods that are easy to digest, such as dry toast and gelatin.

How To Handle Diarrhea

Diarrhea most often begins in the third or fourth week of radiation therapy. Your doctor may suggest you change your diet, prescribe medicine for you, or give you special instructions to help with the problem. Tell the doctor or nurse if these changes are not controlling your diarrhea.

The following changes in your diet also may help:
- Try a clear liquid diet (water, weak tea, apple juice, clear broth, plain gelatin) as soon as diarrhea starts or when you feel that it's going to start.
- Ask your doctor or nurse to advise you about liquids that won't make your diarrhea worse. Apple juice;peach nectar, weak tea, and clear broth are frequent suggestions.
- Avoid foods that are high in fiber or can cause cramps or a gassy feeling such as raw fruits and vegetables, coffee, beans, cabbage, whole grain breads and cereals, sweets, and spicy foods.
- Eat frequent small meals.
- Avoid milk and milk products if they irritate your bowels.
- When the diarrhea starts to improve, try eating small amounts of low-fiber foods such as rice, bananas, applesauce, mashed potatoes, low-fat cottage cheese, and dry toast.
- Be sure your diet includes foods that are high in potassium (bananas, potatoes, apricots), an important mineral that you may lose through diarrhea.

Diet planning is a very important part of radiation treatment of the stomach and abdomen. Keep in mind that these problems will be reduced greatly when treatment is over. In the meantime, try to pack the highest possible food value into even small meals so that you will have enough calories and vital nutrients.

What Side Effects Occur With Radiation Therapy to the Pelvis?

If you are having radiation therapy to any part of the pelvis (the area between your hips), you might have one or more of the digestive problems already described. You also may have some irritation to your bladder. This can cause discomfort or frequent urination. Drinking fluids can help relieve some of your discomfort. Your doctor can prescribe some medicine to deal with these problems.

There are also certain side effects that occur only in the reproductive organs. The effects of radiation therapy on sexual and reproductive functions depend on which organs are treated. Some of the more common side effects for both men and women do not last long after treatment. Others may be long-term or permanent. Before your treatment begins, ask your doctor about possible side effects and how long they might last.

Effects on Fertility

Scientists are still studying how radiation treatment affects fertility. If you are a women in your childbearing years, you should discuss birth control measures with your doctor. It is not a good idea to become pregnant during radiation therapy. Radiation may injure the fetus. In addition, pregnancy, childbirth, and caring for a very young child can add to the physical and emotional stress of having cancer. If you are pregnant before beginning radiation therapy, special steps should be taken to protect the fetus from radiation.

Depending on the radiation dose, women having radiation therapy in the pelvic area may stop menstruating and may have other symptoms of menopause. Treatment also can result in vaginal itching, burning, and dryness. You should report these symptoms to your doctor or nurse, who can suggest treatment.

For men, radiation therapy to an area that includes the testes can reduce both the number of sperm and their effectiveness. This does not mean that conception cannot occur, however. If you're having this type of treatment, discuss your concerns and your birth control measures with your doctor. If you want to father a child and are concerned about reduced fertility, you can look into the option of banking your sperm before treatment.

Sexual Relations

During treatment to the pelvis, some women are advised not to have intercourse. Others may find that intercourse is painful. You most likely will be able to resume having sex within a few weeks after your treatment ends.

Some shrinking of vaginal tissues occurs during radiation therapy. After your radiation therapy is finished your doctor will advise you about sexual intercourse and how to use a dilator, a device that gently stretches the tissues of the vagina.

With most types of radiation therapy, neither men nor women are likely to suffer any change in their ability to enjoy sex. Both sexes, however, may notice a decrease in their level of desire. This is more likely to be due to the stress of having cancer than to the effects of radiation therapy. This effect most likely will go away when the treatment ends, so it should not become a major concern. A booklet on sexuality and cancer is available without charge from your local American Cancer Society office. There are different versions for male and female patients.

FOLLOW-UP CARE

What Does "Follow-up" Mean?

Once your course of radiation therapy is finished it is important to have regular exams to check the results of your treatment. No matter what type of cancer you have had you will need regular checkups and perhaps lab tests and x-rays. The radiation oncologist will want to see you at least once after your treatment ends. The doctor who referred you for radiation therapy will schedule follow-up visits as needed. Follow-up care in addition to checking the results of your treatment might also include more cancer treatment rehabilitation and counseling. Taking good care of yourself is also a part of following through after radiation treatments.

Who Provides Care After Therapy?

Most patients return to the radiation oncologist for regular follow-up visits. Others are referred back to their original doctor to a surgeon or to a **medical oncologist** a doctor who is trained to give chemotherapy (treatment with anti-cancer drugs). Your follow-up care will depend on the kind of cancer you have and on other treatments that you had or may need.

What Other Care Might Be Needed?

Just as every patient is different follow-up care varies. Your doctor will prescribe and schedule the follow-up care that you need. Don't hesitate to ask about the tests or treatments that your doctor orders. Try to learn all the things you should do to take good care of yourself.

Following are some of the questions that you may want to ask your doctor after you have finished your radiation therapy:
- How often do I need to return for checkups?
- Why do I need more x-rays scans blood tests and so on? What will these tests tell us?
- Will I need chemotherapy, surgery, or other treatments?
- How will you know if I'm cured of cancer? What are the chances that it will come back?
- How soon can I go back to my regular activities?
- Work?
- Sexual activity?
- Sports?
- Do I need to take any special precautions?
- Do I need a special diet?
- Should I exercise?
- Can I wear a **prosthesis**?
- How soon can I have reconstructive surgery?

You may want to use the "Notes" page at the back of this booklet to write down other questions and take the list with you to your doctor's office.

What If Pain Is a Problem?

A few patients need help to manage pain if it continues after radiation therapy. You should not use a heating pad or warm compress to relieve pain in any area treated with radiation. Mild pain medicine may be enough for some people. If you have severe pain, ask the doctor about prescription drugs or other methods of relief. Be as specific as possible when telling the doctor about your pain so you can get the best treatment for it. If you are unable to get relief from pain, you may want to talk with a doctor who is a pain specialist.

Because pain can be worse when you are afraid or worried, it may help to try relaxation exercises. Other methods such as hypnosis, biofeedback, and acupuncture may be useful for some cancer patients. *Questions and Answers About Pain Control* is a free booklet that may help you understand more about cancer pain (See Resources.)

How Can I Help Myself After Radiation Therapy?

Patients who have had radiation therapy need to continue some of the special care used during treatment at least for a short while. For instance, you may have skin problems for several weeks after your treatments end. You should continue to be gentle with skin in the treatment area until all signs of irritation are gone. Don't try to scrub off the marks in your treatment area. They will fade and wear away.

You may find that you still need extra rest while your healthy tissues are rebuilding. Keep taking naps as needed and try to get more sleep at night. You may need some time to test your strength, little by little, so you may not want to resume a full schedule of activities right away.

When Should I Call the Doctor?

After treatment for cancer, you're likely to be more aware of your body and to notice even slight changes in how you feel from day to day. The doctor will want you to report any unusual symptoms. If you have any of the problems listed below, tell your doctor at once:

- A pain that doesn't go away, especially if it's always in the same place.
- Lumps, bumps, or swelling.

- Nausea, vomiting, diarrhea, or loss of appetite.
- Unexplained weight loss.
- A fever or cough that doesn't go away.
- Unusual rashes, bruises, or bleeding.
- Any other signs mentioned by your doctor or nurse.

What About Returning to Work?

Many people continue to work during radiation therapy, but if you have stopped working, you can return to your job as soon as you feel up to it, even while your radiation therapy is continuing. If your job requires lifting or heavy physical activity, you may need to change your activities until you have regained your strength.

When you are ready to return to work, it is important to learn about your rights regarding your job and health insurance. If you have any questions about employment issues, contact the Cancer Information Service or the American Cancer Society. They can help you find local agencies that respond to problems cancer survivors sometimes face regarding employment and insurance rights. These organizations are listed in the resources section at the back of this booklet.

CONCLUSION

We hope the information in this booklet will help you understand how radiation therapy is used to treat cancer. Knowing what to expect when you go for your treatments should lessen the anxiety you may be feeling. Don't forget to call on your health care team whenever you need more information.

GLOSSARY

These are words that appear in this booklet or that you may hear your health team use.

Adjuvant therapy: A treatment method used in addition to the primary therapy. Radiation therapy often is used as an adjuvant to surgery.

Alopecia (*al-oh-PEE-she-ah*): Hair loss.

Anesthesia: Loss of feeling or sensation resulting from the use of certain drugs or gases.

Antiemetic (*an-tee-eh-MET-ik*): A medicine to prevent or relieve nausea or vomiting.

Benign tumor: A growth that is not a cancer and does not spread to other parts of the body.

Biological therapy: Treatment by stimulation of the body's immune defense system.

Biopsy: The removal of a sample of tissue to see whether cancer cells are present.

Brachytherapy (*BRAK-ee-THER-ah-pee*): Internal radiation treatment achieved by implanting radioactive material directly into the tumor or very close to it. Sometimes called "internal radiation therapy."

Cancer: A general term for more than 100 diseases that have uncontrolled abnormal growth of cells that can invade and destroy healthy tissues.

Catheter: A thin flexible tube through which fluids enter or leave the body.

Chemotherapy: Treatment with anticancer drugs.

Cobalt 60: A radioactive substance used as a radiation source to treat cancer.

Dietitian (also **registered dietitian**): A professional who plans diet programs for proper nutrition.

Dosimetrist (*do-SIM-uh-trist*): A person who plans and calculates the proper radiation dose for treatment.

Electron beam: A stream of particles that produces high-energy radiation to treat cancer.

External radiation: Radiation therapy that uses a machine located outside of the body to aim high-energy rays at cancer cells.

Fluoride: A chemical applied to the teeth to prevent tooth decay.

Gamma rays: High-energy rays that come from a radioactive source such as cobalt-60.

Gray: A measurement of absorbed radiation (dose; 1 Gray = 100 rads).

High dose rate remote brachytherapy: A type of internal radiation in which each treatment is given in a few minutes while the radioactive source is in place. The source of radioactivity is removed between treatments. Also known as high dose rate remote radiation therapy.

Hyperfractionated radiation: Division of the total dose of radiation into smaller doses that are given more than once a day.

Implant: A small container of radioactive material placed in or near a cancer.

Internal radiation: A type of therapy in which a radioactive substance is implanted into or close to the area needing treatment.

Interstitial radiation: A radioactive source (implant) placed directly into the tissue (not in a body cavity).

Intracavitary radiation: A radioactive source (implant) placed in a body cavity such as the chest cavity or the vagina.

Intraoperative radiation: A type of external radiation used to deliver a large dose of radiation therapy to the tumor bed and surrounding tissue at the time of surgery.

Linear accelerator: A machine that creates high-energy radiation to treat cancers, using electricity to term a stream of fast-moving subatomic particles. Also called megavoltage (MeV) linear accelerator or a linac.

Malignant: Cancerous (see cancer).

Medical oncologist: A doctor who specializes in using chemotherapy to treat cancer.

Metastasis: The spread of a cancer from one part of the body to another. Cells in the second tumor are like those in the original tumor.

Oncologist: A doctor who specializes in treating cancer.

Palliative care: Treatment to relieve, rather than cure, symptoms caused by cancer. Palliative care can help people live more comfortably.

Physical therapist: A health professional trained in the use of treatments such as exercise and massage.

Platelets: Special blood cells that help stop bleeding.

Prosthesis: An artificial replacement of a part of the body.

Rad: Short form for "radiation absorbed dose"; a measurement of the amount of radiation absorbed by tissues (100 rad = 1 Gray).

Radiation: Energy carried by waves or a stream of particles.

Radiation oncologist: A doctor who specializes in using

radiation to treat cancer.

Radiation physicist: A person trained to ensure that the radiation machine delivers the right amount of radiation to the treatment site.

Radiation therapist: A person with special training who runs the equipment that delivers the radiation.

Radiation therapy: The use of high-energy penetrating rays or subatomic particles to treat disease. Types of radiation include x-ray, electron beam, alpha and beta particles, and gamma rays. Radioactive substances include cobalt, radium, iridium, and cesium. (See also gamma rays, brachytherapy, teletherapy, and x-ray.)

Radiologist: A physician with special training in reading diagnostic x-rays and performing specialized x-ray procedures.

Radiotherapy: See radiation therapy.

Remote brachytherapy: See high dose rate remote brachytherapy.

Simulation: A process involving special x-ray pictures that are used to plan radiation treatment so that the area to be treated is precisely located and marked for treatment.

Teletherapy: Treatment in which the radiation source is at a distance from the body. Linear accelerators and cobalt machines are used in teletherapy.

Treatment port or field: The place on the body at which the radiation beam is aimed.

Tumor: An abnormal mass of tissue. Tumors are either benign or malignant.

Unsealed internal radiation therapy: Internal radiation therapy given by injecting a radioactive substance into the bloodstream or a body cavity. This substance is not sealed in a container.

White blood cells: The blood cells that fight infection.

X-ray: High-energy radiation that can be used at low levels to diagnose disease or at high levels to treat cancer.

RESOURCES

Information about cancer is available from the sources listed below. You may wish to check for additional information at your local library or bookstore and from support groups in your community.

Cancer Information Service (CIS)

The Cancer Information Service, a program of the National Cancer Institute, is a nationwide telephone service for cancer patients and their families and friends, the public, and health care professionals. The staff can answer questions and can send booklets about cancer. They also may know about local resources and services. One tollfree number, 1-800-4-CANCER (1-800-422-6237), connects callers with the office that serves their area. Spanish-speaking staff members are available.

PDQ

People who have cancer, those who care about them, and doctors need up-to-date and accurate information about cancer treatment. To meet these needs, PDQ was developed by NCI. PDQ contains an up-to-date list of trials all over the country. The Cancer Information Service, at 1-800-4-CANCER, can provide PDQ information to doctors, patients, and the public.

Publications

Cancer patients, their families and friends, and others may find the following books useful. They are available free of charge by calling 1-800-4-CANCER.
- Chemotherapy and You: A Guide to Self Help During Treatment.
- Eating Hints: Recipes and Tips for Better Nutrition During Cancer Treatment.
- Questions and Answers About Pain Control.
- Taking, Time: Support for People with Cancer and the People Who Care About Them.
- What You Need To Know About Cancer. A series of booklets about different types of cancer; ask for the type of cancer you have.

American Cancer Society (ACS)

The American Cancer Society is a voluntary organization with a national office and local units all over the country. It supports research, conducts educational programs, and offers many services to patients and their families. To obtain information about services and activities in local areas, call the Society's toll-free number, 1-800-ACS-2345 (1-800-227-2345), or the number listed under "American Cancer Society" in the white pages of the telephone book. American Cancer Society 1599 Clifton Road, N.E. Atlanta, GA 30329 1-800-ACS-2345.

Index

INDEX • 155

2'-deoxyribouridine, 15
5-fluoruracil, 15
acute, 8, 15, 51, 130-131
acute myeloid leukemia, 51
adenocarcinoma, 54, 66, 72
adjuvant, 15, 17, 23, 35-36, 38,
  50, 61-64, 71, 73-75, 83, 113,
  147
Adriamycin, 60, 73
African American, 26, 41
alopecia, 15, 51, 91, 113, 133,
  147
American Cancer Society, 11, 13-
  14, 18, 25, 29, 38, 40, 46, 49-
  50, 87, 92, 104-105, 108, 111,
  113, 118, 121, 136, 144, 147,
  151-152
AML, 51
androgens, 52
angiogenesis, 54
animal data, 71
anti-cancer, 15
anti-estrogen, 17
areola, 45, 56
Ashkenazi Jews, 27
axillary, 14, 21-22, 33, 47, 49, 56
benefits, 15-16, 30, 36, 40, 44,
  63, 81, 89, 106, 118-119
benign, 7, 28, 32, 47, 54, 56-57,
  114-115, 148, 150
biopsy, 18, 32-33, 38, 47-48, 56,
  65, 148
birth control pills, 29, 31, 37
blood clots, 37
bone marrow, 22-24, 36-37, 52-
  53, 65, 68, 71-72, 74-77, 88,
  92-94, 114

BRCA1, 18, 26-28, 70
BRCA2, 18, 27-28
breast conserving treatment, 61
Breast Self-Examination, 12, 42,
  54
C-erb, 64
calcium deposits, 47, 56
Canada, 59, 62, 73
carcinogens, 8
cathepsin, 40
chemotherapy, 14-16, 22-24, 34-
  37, 44, 50-51, 53, 57, 59-63,
  67-69, 71-73, 75-76, 81-89, 91-
  108, 110-114, 119, 133, 145,
  148-149, 151
children, 8, 29, 93-94, 128
cholesterol, 36
Clinical Breast Examination, 13,
  54
core biopsy, 47
cranio-caudal, 60
cure, 7, 11, 16-17, 39, 74, 83,
  105, 115, 133, 149
cyst, 32, 47
cytotoxic, 14-15, 65, 67
cytoxan, 15, 73
DCIS, 19, 21, 23, 50, 54, 70
deoxyribonucleic acid, 15
deoxythymidylate, 15
diet, 8, 30-31, 63, 92, 98, 104-
  105, 125-126, 134-135, 142,
  145, 148
diethylstilbestrol, 30
disodium pamidronate, 61, 73
DNA, 15, 39-40, 68
drug resistance, 37

ductal carcinoma in situ, 19, 21, 50, 54, 70
ducts, 11, 21, 31-32, 47, 54-57
endocrine therapy, 14, 16
endometrial cancer, 17, 52
epidemiological studies, 63
estrogen, 16-17, 29, 31, 36, 39, 48, 52, 62, 64, 66-69
Europe, 26, 33, 59-60, 67, 70, 73
false-positive, 27, 37, 41
fine-needle aspiration biopsy, 47
FNAB, 47
Food and Drug Administration, 15, 24, 29, 58, 66
Former Soviet Union, 59, 65
France, 59, 62-63
genetic inheritance, 8
Germany, 59-60
glands, 11, 19, 34, 55, 138
hair loss, 15, 36, 87-88, 91, 113, 131, 133, 147
Halsted, 33-35
heart disease, 8, 31, 69, 75
HER-2 oncogene, 40
High Definition Imaging, 32
Hiroshima, 29
implant placement, 44-45
in situ, 19, 21, 31, 39, 41, 50, 54-56, 66, 70
India, 59, 64-65, 74
inflammatory breast cancer, 23, 31, 39, 55
intraoperative radiation, 16, 119, 124, 149
invasive, 7, 19, 21, 31, 39, 41, 54-55, 66, 72, 76
iridium-192, 72
Italy, 59, 61
Japan, 30, 59, 61, 70, 73
Japanese women, 30
latissimus dorsi, 45
LCIS, 19, 21, 50, 55
leukemia, 15, 51, 112
lobular carcinoma, 19, 21, 50, 55, 66, 70
lobules, 11, 19, 31, 55, 57
local therapy, 14, 47
lumpectomy, 14, 22-23, 34-35, 48-49, 54, 62, 140
lymph nodes, 14, 19-23, 33, 35, 39, 47, 49, 56
malignant, 7, 54, 57, 63-64, 114-115, 149-150
mammography, 18-19, 21, 32, 38, 40-42, 44, 46, 54-56, 60, 66, 70, 73
mastectomy, 14, 21-23, 25, 33-35, 43-45, 48-50, 61, 63, 65, 140
menopausal, 23, 29-30, 38
methotrexate, 15, 68, 71, 73
Mitomycin C, 60
monoclonal antibodies, 53
MQSA, 42
mucinous carcinoma, 56
Nagasaki, 29
National Institutes of Health, 16, 26, 40, 57, 81, 117
nausea, 15, 36-37, 51, 87-91, 101, 104, 110, 114, 137, 141, 147-148
neoadjuvant chemotherapy, 61, 73
neoplasia, 19, 21, 55
neural invasion, 62
nipple, 13, 31-32, 41, 43, 45, 47, 56, 66
nipple discharge, 41, 47
oophorectomy, 52
osteoporosis, 30
overweight, 31
p53, 28, 64, 68, 70, 75
Paget's disease, 31-32, 56, 66
palpable, 32
PBSC, 53
peripheral blood stem cell, 53
phyllodes, 56-57
pregnancy, 11, 13, 29, 51-52, 62, 70, 76, 103, 143
primary ways, 7-8
progesterone, 11, 39, 48
progestins, 52
prostheses, 44
quadrantectomy, 14, 49, 61
radiation therapy, 14, 16, 23, 29, 37, 44, 49, 68, 76, 82-83, 100, 113-115, 117-128, 130-150
radical mastectomy, 14, 22-23, 25, 34, 49, 61, 65
radon, 9

receptors, 17, 39, 48, 62, 64
reconstruction, 21-23, 43-45, 50
rectus abdominus, 45
risks, 15, 29, 40-41, 44, 72, 106, 119
saline implants, 44
scirrhous cancer, 57
secondary ways, 7, 9
side effect, 15, 49, 88, 90-91, 94, 131, 134, 141
silicone gel, 44
Spain, 59, 65
staging, 18, 20, 67
surgery, 14, 21-24, 28, 33-35, 37-39, 41, 43-44, 48-52, 60, 63, 68, 71-74, 76, 82-83, 113, 119-120, 124, 145, 147, 149
surgical biopsy, 48
tamoxifen, 17, 36-37, 52, 57, 64, 67-69, 71, 74-76
tetracycline, 72
thymidylate, 15
TNM, 20
toremifene, 71, 76
tubular carcinomas, 57
tumor suppressor gene, 28
two-step procedure, 33, 48
ultrasound, 18, 32, 47
United Kingdom, 27, 59, 63
United States, 4, 11, 14-15, 30, 34, 42, 59, 62, 65-67, 69, 73
United States of America, 4, 11, 65
unknown factors, 8-9
verapamil, 37
white women, 26, 41
Zofran, 36